Renal Diet Cookbook

125 Recipes Low in Sodium, Potassium, Phosphorus, and Protein for Your Kidney Disease—Complete Guide to Controlling Your CKD and Avoiding Dialysis Included

Benjamin Olivier

Published by Northern Press Inc.

Contents

Introduction

CKD, or chronic kidney disease, affects over thirty million Americans. Only a small fraction of those diagnosed will ever have to face a kidney transplant or dialysis. For more the fifty years, people have known that diet has a large impact on the outcome of CKD patients by slowing the rate of their progression, delaying the onset of their symptoms, decreasing the risk of cardiovascular problems, and improving the internal environment of their body. For those who already suffer from cardiovascular disease, high blood pressure, high cholesterol, or diabetes, dietary changes can go a long way to help stabilize the function of the kidneys and improve survival.

Unfortunately, for most newly diagnosed CKD patients, learning to follow the renal diet can be challenging. This can be even scarier if they have already been told to reduce their sugar intake or fats. The main question most people will have when facing a renal diet is "With all of these restrictions, what can I eat?" They are afraid that they will have to eat boring and bland foods, which makes any diet unsustainable and difficult to follow.

This book is here to help with just that. Managing CKD will require lifestyle changes, but you're not alone. But without knowing what can happen, fear, anxiety, depression, and uncertainty are common among CKD patients. A lot may even feel that dialysis is inevitable, and you could find yourself wondering it's worth your time and effort. Only one in fifty people diagnosed with CKD faces dialysis. With the right tools, you can delay and prevent end-stage renal disease and dialysis. With simple management strategies, you can live a full and productive life.

What It Means to Have CKD

It is going to sound scary when you get diagnosed with chronic kidney disease and you probably have a lot of question. This disease can be managed very well. It will take some exploration, patience, and time to see the big picture. Your first step to managing kidney disease is being able to understand it. Let's take a look at the role your kidneys play in your health, how your diet plays an important role in helping to manage kidney disease, and what happens when you develop kidney disease.

Once you have been diagnosed with CKD, it will be helpful to explore this disease and learn about some normal symptoms. A simple definition is a gradual loss of the function of your kidneys. Because our bodies constantly produce waste, our kidneys play a big role to remove these toxins and keep our system working properly. Tests will be done to measure the level of waste in your blood and figure out how well your kidneys are working. Your doctor will be able to find out the filtration rate of your kidneys and figure out what stage of CKD you are in.

There are five stages that show how the kidneys function. Within the early stages, people won't experience any symptoms, and it is very easy to manage. Oftentimes, kidney disease isn't found until it becomes advanced. Most symptoms don't appear until the toxins build-up in the body from the damage that has been done to the kidneys. This usually happens in the later stages. Changes in how you urinate, vomiting, nausea, swelling, and itching could be caused by decreased ability to filtrate the toxins. This is why an early diagnosis that is critical to positive outcomes can come later when the disease has progressed.

There isn't a cure for CKD, but you can manage this disease. Making changes to your lifestyle and diet can slow down the progression and help you stay away from symptoms that normally start to show up later. These lifestyle changes can improve your total health and allow you to manage other conditions. Once you begin making changes to your daily food habits, you will see improvement in these conditions including diabetes and hypertension.

You can live a happy, healthy, and long life while managing CKD and making changes early can slow down the progression of this disease for years.

How the Kidneys Work

Our kidneys are bean-shaped filters that work in teams. They have a very important job since they keep our bodies stable. They use signals from the body like blood pressure and sodium content to help keep us hydrated and our blood pressure stable.

If the kidneys don't function right, there are numerous problems that could happen. When the filtration of these toxins becomes slow, these harmful chemicals can build up and cause other reactions within the body like vomiting, nausea, and rashes. When the kidney's functions continue to decrease, its ability to get rid of water and release hormones that control blood pressure can also be affected. Symptoms such as high blood pressure or retaining water in your feet might happen. With time having reduced kidney function could cause long-term health problems such as osteoporosis or anemia.

The kidneys work hard, so we have to protect them. They can filter around 120 to 150 quarts of blood each day. This will create between 1 and 2 quarts of urine that are made up of excess fluid and waste products.

Causes

Conditions like hypertension and diabetes have been associated with kidney disease and play key roles in decreasing how these organs function. Let's look at some common causes of CKD and what you need to think about if you have more than one of the following conditions.

❖ Diabetes

This disease changes how your body uses and produces insulin. This hormone gets released from the pancreas that gets sugar from the blood and then sends it to other organs that need it to function properly. If you have been diagnosed with diabetes, there is a chance you know all these information already and you have learned how to manage it with medicine and diet.

If your diabetes is uncontrolled or chronic, it could damage your kidneys, and it is a major factor in developing CKD. Diabetes is the main cause of kidney disease. One of the jobs for kidneys is filtering the fluid in the body and getting rid of the waste along with water that isn't needed. Think about this fluid going through the kidneys constantly 24 hours a day. Normal filtration systems are strong enough to handle all the pressure. If there are large sugar molecules in the blood, this can increase the pressure that is put on the filter and, over time, it will break.

❖ Hypertension/High Blood Pressure

This can cause kidney damage and could be caused by damage to the kidneys. The blood vessels send all the blood through the entire body. This alone puts pressure on the artery walls. If this pressure becomes too high, it might damage the vessel walls, especially the small vessels like the ones found inside the kidneys. The blood vessels that go through the kidneys change molecules during this filtration process. If these walls get damaged, it could hurt how the filtration process works and causes the kidneys to become damaged and, thus, causing CKD.

The kidney's main function is controlling blood pressure by producing hormones. When the kidneys get damaged, they won't be able to regulate these hormones, and your blood pressure could go up. If you struggle to control your hypertension or want to regulate your blood pressure, managing your lifestyle and diet could help. Many elements of a kidney-friendly diet can help manage your hypertension. It is important to think about this as you figure out what changes you want to make for the good of your health.

Treating Chronic Kidney Disease

Being able to manage chronic kidney disease takes a lot of lifestyle changes, dietary modifications, and working with your doctors. You can up your chances for better outcomes by learning about the disease and finding out everything you can about the choices you make. Knowledge is power, so grab everything you can. This is very true with you have chronic kidney disease.

❖ Diet

Learning how to eat with CKD is a bit overwhelming, but with anything that is new, when you begin practicing it, it will soon be a normal part of your life that won't require any thought. The basic guideline is restricting phosphorus, potassium, sodium, protein, and at times, fluids. This is all based on the results of your blood work. Your health care professional and dietitian can make a diet plan specifically for your needs. The rest is totally up to you. How well you comply with restrictions on your diet has a large influence on how fast the disease progresses.

❖ Lifestyle

Just like a diet, the choices you make in life plays a huge part in managing your CKD. Staying away from alcohol, quitting smoking, reducing stress, managing your weight, getting enough sleep, and exercising regularly are all great lifestyle practices. They could help you reduce or manage your risk of chronic diseases like high blood pressure, diabetes, and heart disease. Lifestyle choices that are practiced on a regular basis could make a large difference in the way you feel emotionally and physically.

❖ Health Care Team

Managing and treating your chronic kidney disease needs to involve a good health care team. You should have a dietitian, social workers, nurses, and a renal doctor. These people all give specific expertise. When they work together, they are a professional support system to guide and educate you about your chronic kidney disease. Health care professionals who are experts in renal failure will give you the best information. Make sure they work together to create an individual plan for your specific needs. You have to be honest and open with your team about the way you feel and the diet and lifestyle choices you make for them to help you. They aren't going to judge you but help you make the right choices so you can manage your CKD.

Slowing Down Kidney Disease

Now that you know what CKD is, let's look at how to slow the progress. This information will give you specific steps to do to develop a healthier lifestyle and diet. You have to keep an open mind and take it one step at a time. Having a positive attitude is important and the way you embrace the steps will determine how you manage your kidney disease. With some determination and willpower from you, you will soon be in charge of your destiny and health.

1. Commit

You might begin feeling a bit overwhelmed when you think about this disease. Take a few deep breaths. Everything is going to be fine because you've got this. Just like any life changes, creating new habits will take time. Just take it one day at a time. Start preparing yourself mentally by telling yourself that you can control this disease by managing your lifestyle and diet.

Promise yourself that you will do your best every day to change your lifestyle and habits. Your commitment to yourself and your motivation to follow through will help you manage your kidney disease. Keep in mind that the earlier this disease gets detected, the better you can treat it. There is a goal for your treatment: slowing down the disease and keeping it from getting any worse. This is one good thing about kidney disease: It lets you take control so you can manage it.

2. Know Your Nutritional Needs

There isn't one diet plan that will be right for everybody who has kidney disease. What you are able to eat is going to change with time. It all depends on how well your kidneys function and factors such as being a diabetic. If you can work closely with your health team and constantly learning, you will be able to make healthy choices that will fit your needs. You can manage your disease and be successful.

Here are some basic guidelines that are useful for anyone who has chronic kidney disease:

❖ Protein

Protein is found in plant and animal foods. Protein is a macronutrient that is needed for a healthy body. For people who have chronic kidney disease having too much isn't good. As the function of the kidney's decline, the body doesn't have the ability to get rid of the waste that gets produced when protein gets broken down and it begins to build up in the blood. The correct amount of protein depends on what stage your kidney disease is in, your body size, appetite, levels of albumin, and other factors. A dietitian could help you figure out your daily limits of protein intake. Here is a general guideline to give you an idea of the amount of protein you should be eating: 37 to 41 grams of protein daily.

If you have been diagnosed with CKD and you smoke, you are increasing the risk of developing end-stage renal disease. Smoking harms almost every organ in the body. Stopping might be the most important thing you can do for your body. Talk with your doctor about ways to help you stop.

❖ Fats

When you are going through times where you are having to restrict what you eat, it is good to know that being able to eat healthy fats is another macronutrient that you need to include daily. Eating healthy fats makes sure you are getting all the essential fatty acids that can help your body in many ways. Polyunsaturated and monounsaturated fats are both unsaturated fats but they are healthy fats because of their benefits to the heart like decreasing LDL, increasing HDL, and lowering the total cholesterol levels. The correct types of fat might decrease inflammation within the body and will protect your kidney from more damage. You should try to include small amounts of these fats into your daily diet.

❖ Carbohydrates

Carbs are another macronutrient that the body needs. This is what the body uses for energy. They also give the body many minerals, fiber, and vitamins that help protect the body. The body needs 130 grams of carbs daily for normal function.

❖ Sodium

Consuming too much sodium makes you thirsty. This can cause increased blood pressure and swelling. Having high blood pressure could cause even more damage to the kidneys that are already unhealthy. Consuming less sodium will lower blood pressure and could slow down chronic kidney disease. The normal recommendation for anyone who has CKD is to keep their sodium intake around 2,000 mg daily. To have the best success is remembering that eating fresh is the best. Sodium can be found in all pickled, cured, salted, or processed foods. Fast foods, frozen and canned can also be high in sodium. Foods that are less processed will have the least amount of sodium. If going "fresh is the best" is the lifestyle change you want to do, you will be giving your body a healthy boost.

❖ Potassium

Potassium can be found in many beverages and foods. It has an important role. It regulates the heartbeat and keeps muscles functioning. People who have kidneys that aren't healthy will need to limit their intake of foods that will increase how much potassium is in the blood. It might increase it to dangerous levels. Eating a diet that restricts your level of potassium means eating around 2.000 milligrams each day. Your dietitian or doctor can tell you what level of potassium would be right for you based on your individual needs and blood work.

In order to lessen the buildup of potassium, you have to know what foods are low and high in potassium. This way you know what foods to be careful around.

❖ Phosphorus

Kidneys that are healthy can help the body regulate phosphorus. When you have CKD, your kidneys can't remove excess phosphorus or get rid of it. This results in high levels of phosphorus in the blood and causes the body to pull calcium from bones. This, in turn, will lead the brittle and weak bones. Having elevated levels of calcium and phosphorus could lead to dangerous mineral deposits in the soft tissues of the body. This is called calciphylaxis.

Phosphorus can be found naturally in plant and animal proteins and in larger levels in processed foods. By choosing foods that are low in phosphorus will keep the phosphorus levels in your body safe. The main rule to keep from eating unwanted phosphors goes back to "fresh is the best" concept. Basically stay away from all process foods. Normal phosphorus intake for anyone who has CKD needs to be around 800 to 1,000 milligrams daily.

❖ Supplements and Vitamins

Instead of relying on supplements, you need to follow a balanced diet. This is the best way to get the number of vitamins your body needs each day. Because of the restrictive CKD diet, it can be hard to get the necessary nutrients and vitamins you need. Anyone who has CKD will have greater needs for vitamins that are water soluble. Certain renal supplements are needed to get the needed extra water soluble vitamins. Renal vitamins could be small doses of vitamin C, biotin, pantothenic acid, niacin, folic acid, Vitamins B12, B6, B2, and B1.

The kidney converts inactive vitamin D to an active vitamin D so our bodies can use it. With CKD, kidneys lose the ability to do this. Your health care provider could check your parathyroid hormone, phosphorus, and calcium levels to figure out if you need to take any supplements of active vitamin D. This type of vitamin D requires a prescription.

If your doctor hasn't prescribed a supplement, don't hesitate to ask them if you would benefit from one. To help keep you healthy, only use supplements that have been approved by your dietitian or doctor.

❖ Fluids

A main function for the kidneys is regulating the balance of fluids in the body. For many individuals who have CKD, you don't have to restrict your fluid intake if your output is normal. As the disease progresses, there will be a decline in output and an increase in retention. If this happens, restricting fluids will become necessary. You have to pay attention to how much fluid you are releasing. Let your health care team know if you see that your output is declining. They will be able to tell you how much fluid you should limit on a daily basis to keep healthy fluid levels to prevent an overload of fluid in the body along with other complications that are associated with extra fluid buildup like congestive heart failure, pulmonary edema, edema, and high blood pressure.

3. Understand Your Calorie Requirements

Each person's calorie requirements will be different and it doesn't matter if they do or don't have CKD. If they do have CKD, picking the correct foods and eating the right amount of calories will help your body. Calories give us the energy to function daily. They can help to slow the progression of kidney disease, keep a healthy weight, avoid losing muscle mass, prevent infections. Eating too many calories could cause weight gain, and that can put more of a burden on your kidneys. It is important that you get the correct amount of calories. The amount of calories for a person with CKD is about 60 to 70 calories per pound of body weight. If you weigh about 150 pounds, you need to consume around 2,000 calories per day.

4. Read Food Labels

It takes time to learn the renal diet and make it a part of your life. Lucky for you all packaged foods come with nutrition labels along with an ingredient list. You need to read these labels so you can choose the right foods for your nutrition needs.

The main ingredients you need to look for on the labels are potassium, phosphorus, sodium, and fat. Manufacturers of food are required by law to list the sodium and fat content of the food. They aren't required to list potassium or phosphorus. It is important to find this information in other places like the internet or books.

5. Portion Control

When you have kidney disease, controlling your portions is important. This doesn't mean you have to starve yourself. It doesn't matter what stage of CKD you are in but eating moderately is important when preserving your kidney health. The biggest part is making sure you don't feel deprived. You can enjoy many different foods as long as they are kidney-friendly and don't overeat. When you cut back on foods that could harm your health and you are careful about what you eat, you are learning portion control. Make a habit of limiting specific foods and eating in moderation when following a kidney diet. It just takes having an informed game plan, resolve, and time.

Picking the correct foods is critical to your kidneys. They are counting on you to give them the correct nutrients so they can function their best. This included minerals, vitamins, fats, carbohydrates, and protein. Too much of any one could harm your body and make your kidneys work harder to get rid of the toxins.

One way to use portion control and picking the correct foods is practicing trying to balance your plate. See your plate with half of it vegetables, a quarter of its protein, and the other quarter carbohydrates.

There is quite a bit of information to learn and it is going to take some time to remember it. That is fine. Take some time and commit to learning. Before you know it, you will be an expert. You will know your body, what it needs in order to thrive and keep your kidneys in good health.

Breakfast

Poached Eggs with Butter

Servings: 2

Macros per Serving:

- ➤ 261 Calories
- ➤ 164 mg Sodium
- ➤ 14 g Protein
- ➤ 173 mg Potassium
- ➤ 226 mg Phosphorus

What You Need:

- ➤ Pepper
- ➤ Vinegar
- ➤ Eggs, 4
- ➤ Chopped cilantro, 1 tbsp
- ➤ Unsalted butter, 2 tbsp
- ➤ Chopped parsley, 1 tbsp

What You Do:

1. Place a pan on low heat and melt the butter. Add in the cilantro and parsley. Allow this to cook for around 1 minute, stirring constantly. Set it off the heat and pour in a small bowl.

2. In a small pot, add 3 inches of water and allow this to come to a simmer. Add in a dash of vinegar.

3. Crack one of the eggs into a small bowl. With a spoon, swirl the water to create a whirlpool, and then slowly pour the egg into the

water. With your spoon, help the whites draw over the yolk of the egg. Repeat this for the rest of the eggs. Allow them to cook for about 4 to 7 minutes, depending on how set you want your yolks to be.

4. Using a slotted spoon, take the eggs out and allow to drain for a minute.

5. Serve the eggs with a tablespoon of the herbed butter and a sprinkling of pepper.

Breakfast Tacos

Servings: 4

Macros Per Serving:

➢ 210 Calories
➢ 364 mg Sodium
➢ 9 g Protein
➢ 141 mg Potassium
➢ 120 mg Phosphorus

What You Need:

➢ Tomato salsa, .25 c
➢ Tortillas, 4
➢ Red pepper flakes
➢ Ground cumin, .5 tsp
➢ Eggs, 4
➢ Minced garlic, .5 tsp
➢ Chopped bell pepper, .5
➢ Chopped sweet onion, .5
➢ Olive oil, 1 tsp

What You Do:

1. Warm the oil in a large pan over medium heat.
2. Place the garlic, bell pepper, and onion into the skillet, cooking until soft. This will take around 5 minutes.
3. Add in the red pepper flakes, cumin, and eggs. Scramble the eggs along with the vegetables until they are cooked to your likeness.
4. Divide the eggs evenly between the 4 tortillas. Top each with 1 tablespoon of salsa.
5. Serve and enjoy.

Feta and Bell Pepper Quiche

Servings: 5

Macros Per Serving:

➢ 172 Calories

➢ 154 mg Sodium

➢ 8 g Protein

➢ 122 mg Potassium

➢ 120 mg Phosphorus

What You Need:

➢ Pepper

➢ Chopped basil, 2 tbsp

➢ Low-sodium feta cheese, .25 c

➢ Plain flour, .25 c

➢ Eggs, 4

➢ Unsweetened rice milk, 1 c

➢ Chopped bell pepper, 1

➢ Minced garlic, 1 tsp

➢ Chopped sweet onion, 1 small

➢ Olive oil, 1 tsp plus more

What You Do:

1. Warm your oven to 400° F. Brush a small amount of olive oil into a 9-inch pie pan.
2. Warm the oil in a skillet on medium. Cook the onion and garlic until they become soft.
3. Add in bell pepper and cook for another 3 minutes.

4. Place the vegetables into the pie plate that has been brushed with olive oil.
5. Place the eggs, flour, and rice milk in a medium bowl and combine until smooth. Add in the basil and feta, then sprinkle with pepper. Stir well to combine.
6. Pour eggs over the vegetables in the pie plate.
7. Bake until edges are golden brown and center is just set. This should take about 20 minutes. This can be served cold, room temperature, or hot.

Pumpkin Apple Muffins

Servings: 12

Macros Per Serving:

- 125 Calories
- 8 mg Sodium
- 2 g Protein
- 177 mg Potassium
- 120 mg Phosphorus

What You Need:

- Diced, cored, and peeled apple, .5 c
- Vanilla, 1 tsp
- Egg, 1
- Olive oil, .25 c
- Honey, .25 c
- Pumpkin puree, 1 c
- Phosphorus-free baking powder, 2 tsp
- Wheat bran, 1 c
- Plain flour, 1 c

What You Do:

1. Warm the oven to 350º F. Take a cupcake tin and place a paper liner into each cup.
2. Add baking powder, wheat bran, and flour into a medium bowl. Stir to mix well.
3. Add the vanilla, egg, olive oil, honey, and pumpkin to a small bowl and combine.

4. Mix the pumpkin mixture into the dry ingredients.

5. Add in the apple and stir to combine.

6. Spoon batter into muffin papers. Don't overfill.

7. Bake for 20 minutes. Once over, stick a toothpick in the middle. If it comes out clean, it means they are done.

Bread Pudding with Blueberries

Servings: 6

Macros Per Serving:

- 382 Calories
- 378 mg Sodium
- 11 g Protein
- 170 mg Potassium
- 120 mg Phosphorus

What You Need:

- Blueberries, 2 c
- Sourdough bread cubes, 6 c
- Ground cinnamon, .5 tsp
- Vanilla, 2 tsp
- Eggs, 3
- Honey, .5 c
- Unsweetened rice milk, 3 c

What You Do:

1. Warm your oven to 350° F.
2. Add cinnamon, vanilla, eggs, honey, and rice milk to a large bowl until well-blended.
3. Add in the bread cubes. Allow the bread to soak for 30 minutes.
4. Add in the blueberries. Stir well to combine. Pour into a 13 x 9 baking dish.
5. Bake for 35 minutes. Check to see if it's done by poking it in the center with a toothpick and it comes out clean.

Citrusy Blueberry Muffins

Servings: 12

Macros Per Serving:

- 252 Calories
- 26 mg Sodium
- 4 g Protein
- 107 mg Potassium
- 79 mg Phosphorus

What You Need:

- Blueberries, 2 c
- Phosphorus-free baking powder, 2 tsp
- Lime zest, 1 tsp
- Plain flour, 2 c
- Light sour cream, .5 c
- Lemon zest, 1 tsp
- Unsweetened rice milk, 1 c
- Eggs, 2
- Sugar, 1 c
- Melted coconut oil, .5 c

What You Do:

1. Warm the oven for 400° F. Take a cupcake tin and place paper liners in each cup.
2. Place the sugar and coconut oil into a medium bowl. Using a hand mixer, beat until fluffy. Add in sour cream, rice milk, and eggs. Scrape and continue to mix until well-blended.

3. Add baking powder, lime zest, lemon zest, and flour to a small bowl. Stir together to combine.
4. Mix the flour mixture into the eggs until it just comes together. Add in the blueberries and stir again.
5. Spoon into prepared muffin papers. Don't overfill.
6. Place into the preheated oven and bake for 25 minutes. Check to make sure a toothpick comes out clean when stuck to the muffins.

Oatmeal Pancakes

Servings: 4

Macros Per Serving:

➤ 195 Calories
➤ 60 mg Sodium
➤ 6 g Protein
➤ 92 mg Potassium
➤ 109 mg Phosphorus

What You Need:

➤ Unsalted butter, 1 tbsp, divided
➤ Egg, 1
➤ Unsweetened rice milk, .5 c
➤ Ground cinnamon
➤ Rolled oats, .25 c
➤ Plain flour, 1 c

What You Do:

1. Put cinnamon, oats, and flour into a medium bowl and stir well to combine.
2. Add the egg and milk to the same bowl. Whisk together. Add this to the flour mixture and whisk well to combine.
3. On a large skillet over medium heat, melt the butter.
4. Take .25 cup of the batter and pour it into the skillet. Cook the pancake until edges are firm and there are bubbles on the surface. This should take about 3 minutes.
5. Flip the pancake and cook until golden brown on this side. This will take around 2 more minutes.
6. Continue with the rest of the batter until it is completely used. Adding butter to skillet as needed.
7. Serve pancakes hot.

Asparagus Frittata

Servings: 2

Macros Per Serving:

- 102 Calories
- 46 mg Sodium
- 6 g Protein
- 248 mg Potassium
- 103 mg Phosphorus

What You Need:

- Chopped parsley, .25 c
- Onion powder, .5 tsp
- Eggs, 4
- Pepper
- EVOO, 2 tsp, divided
- Medium trimmed asparagus spears, 10

What You Do:

1. Start by placing your oven to 450° F.
2. Toss the asparagus spears with a teaspoon of oil and season with a bit of pepper. Lay these out on a cookie sheet and bake for 20 minutes. Stir the spears occasionally and allow them to cook until they are tender and browned.
3. Beat the eggs together with the parsley and onion powder. Add pepper to taste.

4. Slice the asparagus into 1-inch pieces and lay them in the bottom of a medium pan. Drizzle in the remaining oil and shake the pan so that everything distributes.

5. Pour the egg mixture over the asparagus and cook them over medium heat. Once the eggs have set up on the bottom and almost set on the top, place a plate and flip over the pan so that the frittata is on the plate, and then carefully slide the frittata back in the pan to cook on the other side. Allow this to continue cooking for 30 more seconds, or until set.

Broccoli Basil Quiche

Servings: 8

Macros Per Serving:

- ➢ 160 Calories
- ➢ 259 mg Sodium
- ➢ 6 g Protein
- ➢ 173 mg Potassium
- ➢ 101 mg Phosphorus

What You Need:

- ➢ Pepper
- ➢ All-purpose flour, 1 tbsp
- ➢ Minced garlic clove
- ➢ Crumbled feta, .5 c
- ➢ Unsweetened rice milk, 1 c
- ➢ Chopped basil, 2 tbsp
- ➢ Beaten eggs, 3
- ➢ Chopped scallions, 2
- ➢ Chopped tomato
- ➢ Finely chopped broccoli, 2 c
- ➢ Frozen pie crust, 1

What You Do:

1. Turn your oven to 425° F.
2. Lay the pie crust out into a pie pan and use a fork to pierce the crust in a few places so that it doesn't rise too much.

3. Allow the crust to bake for about 10 minutes. Remove and lower the temperature of the oven to 325° F.

4. In a medium bowl, combine the flour, garlic, feta, rice milk, basil, eggs, scallions, tomato, and broccoli. Sprinkle in some pepper.

5. Pour the egg mixture into the pie crust. Allow this to bake for 35 to 45 minutes. When you insert a knife in the center, it should come out clean.

6. Allow the quiche to cool for 10 to 15 minutes before you serve.

Avocado Egg Bake

Servings: 2

Macros Per Serving:

- ➤ 242 Calories
- ➤ 88 mg Sodium
- ➤ 9 g Protein
- ➤ 575 mg Potassium
- ➤ 164 mg Phosphorus

What You Need:

- ➤ Chopped parsley, 1 tbsp
- ➤ Pepper
- ➤ Eggs, 2
- ➤ Halved avocado

What You Do:

1. Start by placing the oven to 425° F.
2. Carefully crack one egg in a small bowl, making sure that the yolk doesn't break.
3. Lay the avocado halves on a baking sheet with the cut side up. Pour the egg into the center of one of the avocado halves. Repeat this for the other egg and other avocado half. Sprinkle with some pepper.
4. Bake for 15 minutes, or until the eggs are set to your desired doneness. Remove and sprinkle with the parsley before serving.

Buckwheat Pancakes

Servings: 4

Macros Per Servings:

- 264 Calories
- 232 mg Sodium
- 7 g Protein
- 399 mg Potassium
- 147 mg Phosphorus

What You Need:

- Butter, 2 tbsp
- Vanilla, 1 tsp
- Egg
- Phosphorus-free baking powder, 2 tsp
- Sugar, 1 tbsp
- All-purpose flour, .5 c
- Buckwheat flour, 1 c
- White vinegar, 2 tsp
- Unsweetened rice milk, 1.75 c

What You Do:

1. Mix together the vinegar and rice milk and let it rest for at least 5 minutes.
2. Meanwhile, mix together the two flours together in a large bowl. Mix in the baking powder and sugar.

3. Add the vanilla and egg to the rice milk mixture and stir together. Pour the wet ingredients into the flour mixture. Mix everything together until it just combined.

4. In a large pan over medium heat, melt 1.5 teaspoons of butter. With a quarter measuring cup, scoop out some batter and pour it into the hot pan. Let it cook for 2 to 3 minutes on one side. Small bubbles should start to form on the surface and the edges will start to dry out. Flip, and allow the pancake to cook for another 1 to 2 minutes.

5. Transfer to a plate and continue cooking until you have used up the batter. Add more butter when you need to.

Overnight Oats

Servings: 2

Macros Per Serving:

- 196 Calories
- 63 mg Sodium
- 8 g Protein
- 114 mg Potassium
- 99 mg Phosphorus

What You Need:

- Honey, 2 tsp
- Vanilla, 1 tsp
- Ground flaxseed, 1 tbsp
- Rolled oats, .5 c
- Unsweetened yogurt, .5 c
- Unsweetened rice milk, .75 c

What You Do:

1. Using a medium bowl, mix everything together. Make sure everything is mixed well.
2. Divide the mixture into two jars and cover them.
3. Allow them to refrigerate for at least 4 hours, but it is best if it can sit overnight.

Bulgur Bowl with Walnuts and Strawberries

Servings: 4

Macros Per Serving:

- 190 Calories
- 13 mg Sodium
- 4 g Protein
- 153 mg Potassium
- 66 mg Phosphorus

What You Need:

- Cacao nibs, 4 tbsp (optional)
- Walnut pieces, 4 tbsp
- EVOO, 4 tsp
- Brown sugar, 4 tsp
- Unsweetened rice milk, 4 tbsp
- Sliced strawberries, 1 c
- Bulgur, 1 c

What You Do:

1. Using a small pot, mix together the bulgur with 2 cups of water and allow it to come to a boil. Reduce the heat so that it simmers, covered, for 12 to 15 minutes. The bulgur should become tender. Set this off the heat and drain off any excess water.
2. Divide the bulgur between 4 bowls and top each with a quarter cup of strawberries, a tablespoon of cacao nibs, a tablespoon of walnut pieces, a teaspoon of olive oil, and a teaspoon of brown sugar.

Open-Face Breakfast Sandwich

Servings: 2

Macros Per Serving:

- 156 Calories
- 195 mg Sodium
- 5 g Protein
- 163 mg Potassium
- 98 mg Phosphorus

What You Need:

- Microgreens, 1 c
- Pepper
- Red onion, 2 slices
- Tomato, 2 slices
- Cream cheese, 2 tbsp, divided
- Halved multigrain bagel

What You Do:

1. Place the bagel halves in a toaster or an oven and allow them to toast lightly.
2. Spread a tablespoon of cream cheese on each half and top with a slice of tomato and 2 rings of onion. Season with a bit of pepper. Top each with half of the microgreens and enjoy.

Peach Berry Parfait

Servings: 2

Macros per Serving:

- 191 Calories
- 40 mg Sodium
- 12 g Protein
- 327 mg Potassium
- 189 mg Phosphorus

What You Need:

- Walnut pieces, 2 tbsp
- Blueberries, .5 c
- Diced small peach
- Vanilla, 1 tsp
- Unsweetened yogurt, 1 c, divided

What You Do:

1. Using a small bowl, combine the vanilla and yogurt. Place 2 tablespoons of yogurt, each in two cups. Divide the fruit between the two cups and top them with the rest of the yogurt.
2. Sprinkle the tops with a tablespoon of walnut pieces each.

Breakfast Soup

Macros Per Serving:

- ➤ 221 Calories
- ➤ 170 mg Sodium
- ➤ 5 g Protein
- ➤ 551 mg Potassium
- ➤ 58 mg Phosphorus

What You Need:

- ➤ Pepper
- ➤ Ground turmeric, 1 tsp
- ➤ Low-sodium broth, 2 c
- ➤ Ground coriander, 1 tsp
- ➤ Halved avocado
- ➤ Ground cumin, 1 tsp
- ➤ Spinach, 2 c

What You Do:

1. With a blender and food processor, add in the turmeric, cumin, coriander, broth, avocado, and spinach. Process the mixture until smooth.
2. Pour the soup into a pot and allow it to heat through for about 2 to 3 minutes. Season to taste with some pepper.

Poultry and Meats

Marinated Pork Tenderloin

Servings: 8

Macros Per Serving:

- 192 Calories
- 151 mg Sodium
- 24 g Protein
- 472 mg Potassium
- 283 mg Phosphorus

What You Need:

- Pork tenderloin, 2 lb
- Dijon mustard, 2 tbsp
- Pepper, .5 tsp
- Minced thyme leaves, 1 tbsp
- Lemon juice, 2 lemons
- Minced garlic, 3 cloves
- EVOO, 4 tbsp, divided

What You Do:

1. Using a small bowl, combine the pepper, thyme, lemon juice, mustard, garlic, and 2 tablespoons of olive oil until well combined.
2. Place the pork tenderloin in a bowl or bag and add in the marinade. Refrigerate the pork for at least 2 hours, but overnight is best.
3. Heat your oven to 400° F.

4. Using an oven-safe skillet, heat it up on medium-high and mix in the rest of the oil. Take the pork tenderloin out of the marinade and lay it into the heated skillet. Allow the tenderloin to sear on all sides.
5. Slide into the oven and allow it to bake for 30 minutes. The juices should run clear. Remove and tent with foil, allowing it to rest for 10 minutes. Slice the tenderloin into half-inch thick slices and serve.

Chicken, Pasta, and Broccoli Casserole

Servings: 6

Macros Per Serving:

- ➢ 351 Calories
- ➢ 152 mg Sodium
- ➢ 24 g Protein
- ➢ 402 mg Potassium
- ➢ 271 mg Phosphorus

What You Need:

- ➢ Shredded cheddar, .25 c
- ➢ Shredded cooked chicken breast, 3 c
- ➢ Unsweetened rice milk, .75 c
- ➢ Pepper
- ➢ Low-sodium chicken stock, 1.5 c
- ➢ All-purpose flour, .25 c
- ➢ Chopped sweet onion, .5
- ➢ Butter, 2 tbsp
- ➢ Packaged broccoli florets, 10 oz
- ➢ Egg noodles, 8 oz

What You Do:

1. Start by placing the oven to 350° F. Grease a two-quart baking dish.
2. Bring a large pot of water to a boil. Add in the egg noodles and let them cook for 5 minutes. Stir in the broccoli, and cook for an additional 3 to 5 minutes until the noodles become tender and the broccoli is fork-tender. Drain off the water and set aside.

3. In a medium pot, add the butter and heat on medium-high and mix in the onion. Sauté for 3 to 5 minutes or until it starts to soften. Stir in the flour and mix until everything is thoroughly combined. Pour in the broth and sprinkle in some pepper. This should simmer for 5 minutes until it starts to thicken. Add in the rice milk and let it cook until heated through.

4. Add the sauce over the noodle mixture and toss everything together. Stir in the cooked chicken and pour into the casserole dish. Sprinkle over the cheddar cheese.

5. Bake the casserole for 20 minutes, uncovered until it has browned up and is bubbling.

Asian-Style Pan-Fried Chicken

Servings: 4

Macros Per Serving:

- ➢ 198 Calories
- ➢ 119 mg Sodium
- ➢ 17 g Protein
- ➢ 218 mg Potassium
- ➢ 148 mg Phosphorus

What You Need:

- ➢ Lemon, cut into wedges
- ➢ Canola oil, 3 tsp, divided
- ➢ Cornstarch, .5 c
- ➢ Low-sodium soy sauce, 1 tsp
- ➢ Minced ginger, 1-inch piece
- ➢ Dry rice wine, 1 tsp
- ➢ Boneless, skinless chicken thighs, 12 oz

What You Do:

1. Mix together the soy sauce, ginger, rice wine, and chicken. Toss everything together and allow it to marinate for 15 minutes.
2. Toss the chicken one more time and then drain off the liquid. One at a time, dip the chicken pieces into the cornstarch so that they are coated.
3. Heat 1.5 teaspoons of oil on medium-high in a medium skillet. Add in half of the chicken to the skillet and cook until it has turned golden brown on one side, around 3 to 5 minutes. Turn the chicken

over and continue to cook until the chicken has cooked through and browned. Place on a plate lined with paper towel to cool and to absorb the excess oil. Add in the remaining oil and cook the rest of the chicken thighs.

4. Serve the chicken with a garnish of lemon.

Curried Chicken and Cauliflower

Servings: 6

Macros Per Serving:

- ➤ 175 Calories
- ➤ 77 mg Sodium
- ➤ 16 g Protein
- ➤ 486 mg Potassium
- ➤ 152 mg Phosphorus

What You Need:

- ➤ Lime juice, 2 limes
- ➤ Dried oregano, .5 tsp
- ➤ Cauliflower head cut into florets
- ➤ EVOO, 4 tsp, divided
- ➤ Bone-in chicken thighs, 6
- ➤ Pepper, .5 tsp, divided
- ➤ Paprika, .25 tsp
- ➤ Ground cumin, .5 tsp
- ➤ Curry powder, 3 tbsp

What You Do:

1. Mix a quarter of a teaspoon of pepper, paprika, cumin, and curry powder in a small bowl.
2. Add the chicken thighs to a medium bowl and drizzle them with 2 teaspoons of olive oil and sprinkle in the curry mixture. Toss them together so that the chicken is well-coated. Cover this up and refrigerate it for at least 2 hours.

3. Place your oven to 400° F.

4. Toss the cauliflower, remaining oil, and the oregano together in a medium bowl. Arrange the cauliflower and chicken across a baking sheet in one layer.

5. Allow this to bake for 40 minutes. Stir the cauliflower and flip the chicken once during the cooking time. The chicken should be browned and the juices should run clear. The temperature of the chicken should reach 165.

6. Serve with some lime juice.

Chicken Breast and Bok Choy

Servings: 4

Macros Per Serving:

- 164 Calories
- 356 mg Sodium
- 24 g Protein
- 187 mg Potassium
- 26 mg Phosphorus

What You Need:

- Lemon, 4 slices
- Pepper
- Boneless, skinless chicken breasts, 4
- Dijon mustard, 1 tbsp
- Thinly sliced small leek
- Julienned carrots, 2
- Thinly sliced bok choy, 2 c
- Chopped thyme, 1 tbsp
- EVOO, 1 tbsp

What You Do:

1. Start by placing the oven to 425° F.
2. Mix together the thyme, olive oil, and mustard in a small bowl.
3. Take 4 18-inch long pieces of parchment paper and fold them in half. Cut them like you would make a heart. Open each of the pieces and lay them flat.

4. In each parchment piece, place .5 cup of bok choy, a few slices of leek, and a small handful of carrots. Lay the chicken breast on top and season with some pepper.

5. Brush the chicken breasts with marinade and top each one with a slice of lemon.

6. Fold the packets up, and roll down the edges to seal the packages.

7. Allow them to cook for 20 minutes. Let them rest of 5 minutes, and make sure you open them carefully when serving.

Baked Herbed Chicken

Servings: 6

Macros Per Serving:

➢ 226 Calories
➢ 120 mg Sodium
➢ 16 g Protein
➢ 158 mg Potassium
➢ 114 mg Phosphorus

What You Need:

➢ Pepper, .25 tsp
➢ Bone-in chicken thighs, 6
➢ Chopped oregano, 1 tbsp
➢ Lemon zest, 1 tsp
➢ Chopped parsley, 1 tbsp
➢ Minced garlic, 4 cloves
➢ Room-temperature butter, 4 tbsp

What You Do:

1. Start by placing your oven to 425° F.
2. Add the lemon zest, parsley, oregano, garlic, and butter to a small bowl and mix well, making sure that everything is distributed evenly throughout the butter.
3. Lay the chicken on a baking pan and gently pull the skin back, but leaving it attached. Brush the thigh meat with some of the butter mixture and lay the skin back over the meat. Sprinkle on some pepper.
4. Bake the chicken for 40 minutes. The skin should be crispy and the juices should be clear. The chicken should reach 165. Allow the chicken to rest for 5 minutes before serving.

Chicken Chow Mein

Servings: 6

Macros Per Serving:

- ➤ 342 Calories
- ➤ 289 mg Sodium
- ➤ 13 g Protein
- ➤ 308 mg Potassium
- ➤ 169 mg Phosphorus

What You Need:

- ➤ Mung bean sprouts, 1 c
- ➤ Chow mein noodles, 10 oz, cooked according to package
- ➤ Low-sodium soy sauce, 1 tsp
- ➤ Diced scallions, 4
- ➤ Canola oil, 2 tsp
- ➤ Julienned carrot
- ➤ Shredded green cabbage, 2 c
- ➤ Sugar, 1 tsp
- ➤ Boneless, skinless sliced chicken thighs, 8 oz
- ➤ Minced garlic, 3 cloves
- ➤ Sesame oil, 1 tsp
- ➤ Cornstarch, 2 tsp
- ➤ Rice wine, 1 tsp
- ➤ Water, 1 tbsp

What You Do:

1. Mix the soy sauce, water, and cornstarch together. Mix in the sesame oil, sugar, and rice wine. Set the mixture to the side.
2. In a wok or a large pan, heat the canola oil.
3. Cook the garlic until it becomes fragrant, stirring it constantly. Mix in the chicken and allow it to cook for a minute, stirring to make sure it browns all over. The chicken won't be cooked through at this point.
4. Add in the scallions, carrot, and cabbage and let them cook for a couple of minutes. The cabbage should begin to silt and the chicken should be cooked through.
5. Add in the noodles and toss everything together. Pour the sauce in and stir everything to coat. Add in the bean sprouts and stir everything together. Set off the heat and enjoy.

Chicken and Cabbage Stir-Fry

Servings: 4

Macros Per Serving:

- 96 Calories
- 156 mg Sodium
- 15 g Protein
- 140 mg Potassium
- 15 mg Phosphorus

What You Need:

- Pepper
- Water, .25 c
- Garlic powder, .5 tsp
- Cornstarch, 1 tbsp
- Thinly sliced green cabbage, 3 c
- Ground ginger, 1 tsp
- Thinly sliced boneless, skinless chicken breast, 10 oz
- Canola oil, 1 tsp

What You Do:

1. Add the oil to a large skillet and heat. Add in the chicken and cook well, stirring often until it is cooked through and browned.
2. Add the cabbage into the skillet and cook for another 2 to 3 minutes. The cabbage should become tender, but it should still be green and crisp.
3. In a separate bowl, combine the water, garlic, ginger, and cornstarch. Pour this into the skillet and cook everything until the sauce has thickened up about 1 minute. Season with some pepper.

Chicken Kebab Sandwich

Servings: 4

Macros Per Serving:

- 217 Calories
- 339 mg Sodium
- 22 g Protein
- 231 mg Potassium
- 80 mg Phosphorus

What You Need:

- Shredded lettuce, 1 c
- Sliced cucumber
- White flatbreads, 4
- Unsweetened yogurt, .25 c
- Pepper
- Minced garlic, 4 cloves, divided
- EVOO, 1 tbsp
- Lemon juice, 2 tbsp
- Boneless, skinless chicken breast, 12 oz

What You Do:

1. Add the lemon juice, half of the garlic, olive oil, and the chicken breast to a medium bowl and toss everything to coat. Season with some pepper and set to the side to marinate while you get the other ingredients ready.
2. Mix the remaining garlic into the yogurt. Season with some pepper, and set to the side.

3. Heat up a pan and add in the chicken with its marinade. Let it cook for 5 minutes until the chicken has browned on the underside. Flip the chicken and continue to cook until it has browned and the juices run clear. Take the chicken out of the pan and allow it to rest for five minutes. Slice up the chicken.

4. In each flatbread, add chicken, cucumber, and lettuce. Top each with the yogurt, and enjoy.

Seafood

Roasted Salmon with Gremolata

Servings: 4

Macros Per Serving:

- 170 Calories
- 55 mg Sodium
- 23 g Protein
- 626 mg Potassium
- 236 mg Phosphorus

What You Need:

- Pepper
- Skinless salmon fillets, 1 lb
- Chopped thyme, 1 tbsp
- Minced garlic, 2 cloves
- Chopped rosemary, 1 tbsp
- Zest and juice of a lemon
- Loosely packed chopped parsley, .5 c

What You Do:

1. Place your oven to 400° F.
2. Mix together the thyme, rosemary, garlic, lemon juice, lemon zest, and parsley in a small bowl.
3. Press the salmon into the herb mixture to coat them on one side. Lay the salmon on a baking pan, herb side up. Sprinkle on some pepper. Bake them for 12 minutes. The fish should flake easily with a fork.

Lime Haddock

Servings: 4

Macros Per Serving:

- ➢ 124 Calories
- ➢ 59 mg Sodium
- ➢ 17 g Protein
- ➢ 283 mg Potassium
- ➢ 176 mg Phosphorus

What You Need:

- ➢ Chopped dill, 2 tsp
- ➢ Crushed almonds, 3 tbsp
- ➢ Olive oil, 1 tbsp
- ➢ Thinly sliced lime, 3
- ➢ Olive oil cooking spray
- ➢ Pepper
- ➢ Haddock fillet, 4, 3 ounce

What You Do:

1. Warm your oven to 400° F.
2. Make sure the haddock is completely dry by patting it with paper towels. Lightly sprinkle with pepper.
3. Lightly spray a 9-inch casserole dish with nonstick spray.
4. Take the lime slices and lay them on the bottom of the baking dish. Lay the haddock on the lime.
5. Brush the olive oil onto the haddock and sprinkle the almonds on top.
6. Allow this to bake until almonds are golden and haddock is cooked through. This should take about 10 minutes.
7. Sprinkle the dill on top.

Orange Shrimp

Servings: 4

Macros Per Serving:

- ➢ 140 Calories
- ➢ 130 mg Sodium
- ➢ 18 g Protein
- ➢ 329 mg Potassium
- ➢ 196 mg Phosphorus

What You Need:

- ➢ Pepper
- ➢ Orange segments, .5 c
- ➢ Unsalted butter, 1 tsp
- ➢ Broccoli florets, 1 c
- ➢ Deveined and peeled shrimp, 12 oz
- ➢ Olive oil, 1 tsp
- ➢ Orange zest, .25 tsp
- ➢ Cornstarch, .5 tsp
- ➢ Orange juice, .5 c

What You Do:

1. Place the orange zest, cornstarch, and orange juice into a small bowl. Set to the side.
2. Place a large pan on medium heat and heat up the oil. Place the shrimp into the warmed skillet and cook until opaque. This will take about 5 minutes. Place cooked shrimp onto a plate. Place the

broccoli into the skillet. Continue cooking until broccoli is tender. Put this on the plate with the shrimp.

3. Pour the orange juice into the skillet and whisk until sauce is glossy and thickened. This will take about 3 minutes.

4. Add in butter while whisking. Place the broccoli, shrimp, and orange segments in the skillet.

5. Toss everything to combine. Sprinkle with pepper.

6. Serve and enjoy.

Herbed Scallops

Servings: 4

Macros Per Serving:

- 131 Calories
- 136 mg Sodium
- 14 g Protein
- 268 mg Potassium
- 176 mg Phosphorus

What You Need:

- Chopped chives, 1 tsp
- Lemon juice, 2 tbsp
- Pepper
- Chopped parsley, 1 tsp
- Sea scallops, 12 oz
- Chopped thyme, 1 tsp
- Olive oil, 1 tbsp

What You Do:

1. Place a large pan with the oil over medium heat.
2. Make sure the scallops are completely dry by patting them with paper towels. Sprinkle them with pepper and place them in the warmed skillet.
3. Sear the scallops, turn over until browned and cooked through. This will take about 4 minutes.
4. Add in chives, thyme, parsley, and lemon juice. Stir to combine.
5. Carefully turn the scallops in the sauce to coat.
6. Serve immediately.

Almond Sole

Servings: 4

Macros Per Serving:

- 113 Calories
- 70 mg Sodium
- 17 g Protein
- 327 mg Potassium
- 168 mg Phosphorus

What You Need:

- Olive oil, 1 tsp
- Chopped parsley, 1 tbsp
- Almond flour, 3 tbsp
- Pepper
- Chopped thyme, 1 tsp
- Sole fillets, 4, 3 oz

What You Do:

1. Preheat oven to 350° F. Line a baking sheet with parchment.
2. Make sure the sole is completely dry by patting them with paper towels.
3. Sprinkle the sole fillets with pepper.
4. Place thyme, parsley, and almond flour into a shallow bowl and mix until blended.
5. Brush the sole with olive oil. Dredge with the almond flour.
6. Put the sole onto the baking sheet.
7. Allow this to bake for 15 minutes or until the sole is opaque.
8. Serve immediately.

Garlic Butter Tilapia

Servings: 4

Macros Per Serving:

➢ 219 Calories

➢ 45 mg Sodium

➢ 17 g Protein

➢ 252 mg Potassium

➢ 149 mg Phosphorus

What You Need:

➢ Pepper

➢ Tilapia fillets, 4, 3 oz

➢ Olive oil, 1 tbsp

➢ Plain flour, 1 tbsp

➢ Zest and juice of .5 lemon

➢ Minced garlic, 1 tsp

➢ Chopped parsley, 2 tbsp

➢ Minced shallot, 1

➢ Melted unsalted butter, .25 c

What You Do:

1. Preheat oven to 400° F. Make sure the tilapia is completely dry by patting it with paper towels.
2. Put flour, parsley, lemon zest, garlic, lemon juice, shallot, and butter in a small bowl and mix well. Set aside.
3. Add oil in an oven-safe large skillet over medium heat.

4. Sprinkle the pepper on the fillets. Place the tilapia into the skillet and brown the tilapia. Turn it once. This should take no more than 4 minutes.

5. Pour the butter mixture over the tilapia and put the skillet into the oven. Bake until just turning opaque in the middle. This will take around 4 minutes.

6. Remove from oven and place on plates. Serve with some sauce from the skillet.

Salmon in Foil

Servings: 4

Macros Per Serving:

- ➤ 119 Calories
- ➤ 29 mg Sodium
- ➤ 13 g Protein
- ➤ 341 mg Potassium
- ➤ 183 mg Phosphorus

What You Need:

- ➤ Peeled and grated ginger, 2 tsp
- ➤ Juice from one lemon
- ➤ Salmon fillet, 4, 2 oz
- ➤ Chopped scallion, 1
- ➤ Asparagus spears, 8
- ➤ Sliced bell pepper, 1
- ➤ Bean sprouts, 2 c

What You Do:

1. Preheat oven to 400° F. Cut 4 pieces of foil that are about one foot squared.
2. Cut the asparagus into 2-inch pieces.
3. Divide out the scallion, asparagus, bell pepper, and bean sprouts evenly across the foil pieces.
4. Put one salmon fillet on top of each vegetable pile.
5. Add ginger and lemon juice into a small bowl and stir to combine. Cover the salmon with this mixture.
6. Fold the foil over the salmon and seal each packet and put them on the baking sheet.
7. Allow this to bake until fish flakes easily. This will take about 20 minutes.
8. Serve immediately.

Salmon Burgers

Servings: 4

Macros Per Serving:

- ➤ 224 Calories
- ➤ 209 mg Sodium
- ➤ 25 g Protein
- ➤ 499 mg Potassium
- ➤ 304 mg Phosphorus

What You Need:

- ➤ Greens or buns, for serving
- ➤ EVOO, 1 tbsp
- ➤ Coarse bread crumbs, .5 c, divided
- ➤ Sliced scallions, 2
- ➤ Pepper
- ➤ Lemon juice, 1 tbsp
- ➤ Zest of a lemon
- ➤ Dijon mustard, 1 tbsp
- ➤ Boneless, skinless salmon, 1 lb

What You Do:

1. Take out the pin bones from the salmon and cut it into chunks. Add half of the salmon to a food processor and mix until it becomes pasty. Mix in the pepper, lemon juice, lemon zest, and mustard. Mix everything together.
2. Transfer this mixture to a bowl and stir in the scallions and a quarter cup of bread crumbs. Form into 4 patties. Lay the rest of the bread

crumbs on a plate and press the patties into the crumbs to coat them.

3. Add the oil to a large pan and heat up. Place the burgers in the pan and cook for 3 to 4 minutes. Flip them over and cook for another 2 to 3 minutes. Serve the patters on a hamburger but or over a bed of greens.

Salmon and Kale

Servings: 4

Macros Per Serving:

➢ 201 Calories
➢ 144 mg Sodium
➢ 26 g Protein
➢ 614 mg Potassium
➢ 332 mg Phosphorus

What You Need:

➢ Dry white wine, .25 c
➢ Sliced lemon
➢ Thyme sprigs, 4
➢ Rosemary sprigs, 4
➢ Paprika .5 tsp
➢ Salmon fillets, 1 lb
➢ Pepper
➢ Sliced small zucchini, 2
➢ Thinly sliced kale leaves, 2 c

What You Do:

1. Start by placing the oven to 450° F.
2. Slice 4 pieces of parchment paper. They should be about 12 inches long.
3. On each of the pieces of parchment, place a half of a cup of kale leaves. Top this with a few slices of zucchini and then sprinkle with some pepper.

4. Place a salmon fillet in each piece of parchment. Season the salmon with paprika and top with a sprig of rosemary and thyme and a slice of lemon. Pour a tablespoon of white wine over each fillet.

5. Fold up the parchment paper and roll the edges together to seal.

6. Bake the packages for 15 minutes. Let them cool for 5 minutes before you open them carefully.

Oven-Fried Fish with Pineapple Salsa

Servings: 4

Macros Per Serving:

- 242 Calories
- 83 mg Sodium
- 27 g Protein
- 474 mg Potassium
- 238 mg Phosphorus

What You Need:

- For the Salsa:
- Chopped cilantro, .25 c
- Lime juice, .5 lime
- Seeded and diced jalapeno, .5 pepper
- Diced red onion, .25 c
- Diced pineapple, 1 c
- For the Fish:
- Butter, 1 tbsp
- Unsweetened rice milk, 2 tbsp
- Beaten egg
- All-purpose flour, .25 c
- Yellow cornmeal, .25 c
- Paprika, .5 tsp
- Garlic powder, .5 tsp
- Whitefish fillets, 1 lb

What You Do:

1. Mix all of the salsa ingredients together in a bowl. Place to the side while you fix the fish.
2. Preheat oven to 400° F and grease a baking dish with the butter.
3. Rub the fish fillets with paprika and garlic powder.
4. Combine the flour and cornmeal.
5. In a separate bowl, mix the egg and milk together.
6. Dip the fish into the egg mixture and then coat them with the flour mixture. Lay the fish in the prepared dish.
7. Bake the fish for 20 minutes. Flip them once, halfway through the cooking process. The fish should be golden and flake easily with a fork.
8. Serve the fish with the pineapple salsa on top.

White Fish and Broccoli Curry

Servings: 6

Macros Per Serving:

➢ 223 Calories

➢ 134 mg Sodium

➢ 18 g Protein

➢ 490 mg Potassium

➢ 194 mg Phosphorus

What You Need:

➢ For the Curry Paste:

➢ EVOO, 2 tbsp

➢ Cumin seeds, .5 tsp

➢ Chopped cilantro stems, .25 c

➢ The tender bottom portion of a lemongrass stalk, chopped

➢ Chopped ginger, 1-inch piece

➢ Turmeric powder, 1 tsp

➢ Chopped medium red chili

➢ Chopped sweet onion, .5

➢ For the Curry:

➢ Sugar, 1 tsp

➢ Juice of a lime

➢ Broccoli florets, 3 c

➢ Tilapia fillet, 1 lb

➢ Cream cheese, .5 c

➢ Unsweetened rice milk, .75 c

What You Do:

1. With a blender or a mortar and pestle, combine the olive oil, cumin seeds, turmeric, cilantro, lemongrass, ginger, chili, and onion. Mix until smooth.

2. For the curry: Add the curry paste to a large skillet and heat to medium-high. Stir occasionally, cooking for 2 to 3 minutes or until it becomes fragrant. Add in the rice milk, stirring until combined. Bring this to a light simmer.

3. Meanwhile, in a small bowl, add the cream cheese and a few tablespoons of the rice-milk mixture. Mix together until blended.

4. Add the broccoli and the tilapia to the skillet, then pour in the cream cheese mixture. Stir everything together until well-blended.

5. Cook this for 3 to 5 minutes or until your fish is cooked. The broccoli should be fork-tender, and the curry is bubbling. Mix in the sugar and the lime juice. Set it off the heat, and serve over white rice.

Lemon Garlic Halibut

Servings: 4

Macros Per Serving:

➢ 169 Calories
➢ 79 mg Sodium
➢ 21 g Protein
➢ 528 mg Potassium
➢ 272 mg Phosphorus

What You Need:

➢ Chopped parsley, 2 tbsp
➢ Zest of a lemon
➢ Skin removed halibut fillets, 1 lb
➢ Pepper
➢ Chopped cilantro, 2 tbsp
➢ Minced garlic, 2 cloves
➢ EVOO, 2 tbsp, divided
➢ Lemon juice, .25 c

What You Do:

1. Set your oven to 400° F.
2. Mix together the garlic, lemon juice, a tablespoon of olive oil, and some pepper. Add the halibut to the bowl and flip it around to make sure that it is coated well. Let this marinate for 10 minutes.
3. Lay the fillets on a baking pan and brush some more of the marinade over the top. Let the fish bake for 12 to 15 minutes. You can brush the fish with the marinade halfway through the cooking process. The fish is done when it can be flaked easily with a fork. Discard any of the leftover marinade.
4. Serve the fish with some parsley, cilantro, and lemon zest.

Creamy Shrimp Fettuccine

Servings: 4

Macros Per Serving:

- 379 Calories
- 527 mg Sodium
- 20 g Protein
- 141 mg Potassium
- 233 mg Phosphorus

What You Need:

- Lemon wedges
- Chopped parsley, 2 tbsp
- Pepper
- Parmesan, .25 c
- Garlic powder, 1 tsp
- Unsweetened rice milk, 1 c
- All-purpose flour, 2 tbsp
- Minced garlic, 3 cloves
- Deveined and peeled shrimp, 10 oz
- EVOO, 2 tbsp, divided
- Dried fettuccine, 8 oz

What You Do:

1. Bring a large pot of salted water up to a boil. Add in the fettuccine and cook them, stirring occasionally until they become al dente. Drain.

2. Add a tablespoon of oil to a pan and heat. Place in the shrimp and cook, stirring occasionally. Cook for 3 to 5 minutes. They should become pink and opaque. With a slotted spoon, take the shrimp out of the pan and place to the side.

3. Add in the rest of the oil. Cook the garlic until fragrant. Add in the flour and mix together, until it creates a paste.

4. Pour the rice milk in slowly, whisking constantly, until the mixture is smooth and all of the rice milk has been added. Mix in the garlic. Lower the heat and simmer for 3 to 4 minutes. The sauce should thicken. Stir in some pepper and the parmesan.

5. Add the noodles to the sauce and mix to coat. Mix in the shrimp and garnish with a lemon wedge and parsley.

Shrimp Fried Rice

Servings: 6

Macros Per Serving:

- 217 Calories
- 431 mg Sodium
- 13 g Protein
- 157 mg Potassium
- 226 mg Phosphorus

What You Need:

- Cooked rice, 3 c
- Sugar snap peas, 1 c
- Deveined and peeled shrimp, 1 lb
- Minced garlic, 3 cloves
- Minced ginger, 2-inch piece
- Chopped sweet onion, .5
- EVOO, 1 tbsp

What You Do:

1. Over medium heat, add oil in a wok or a large pan.
2. Place in the onion and stir constantly for around 3 to 5 minutes. The onion should soften.
3. Add in the garlic and ginger, and stir the mixture until it becomes fragrant.
4. Add in the shrimp and cook until the shrimp has turned opaque and is almost cooked through about 5 minutes.
5. Mix in the rice and snap peas, stirring until everything is well mixed and heated through. Enjoy.

Shrimp and Bok Choy

Servings: 4

Macros Per Serving:

- 92 Calories
- 484 mg Sodium
- 12 g Protein
- 162 mg Potassium
- 217 mg Phosphorus

What You Need:

- Thinly sliced scallions, 2
- Lime juice, 2 tbsp
- Thinly sliced bok choy, 1 lb
- Rice vinegar, 2 tbsp
- Honey, 2 tsp
- Minced ginger, 2-inch piece
- Minced garlic, 3 cloves
- Toasted sesame oil, 1 tsp
- Deveined and peeled shrimp, 12 oz
- Chopped cilantro, .25 c
- Thinly sliced jalapeno pepper

What You Do:

1. Set your oven to 375° F.
2. Mix together the ginger, garlic, and shrimp in a small bowl.
3. In a separate bowl, mix together the rice vinegar, honey, lime juice, and sesame oil.

4. Cut out 4 large circles from parchment paper. It should be at least 12 inches in diameter. On each circle, place a handful of bok choy and top with the shrimp and the garlic mixture, jalapeno slices, and scallions. Drizzle each with a quarter of the lime mixture.

5. Fold up the parchment paper and roll the edges together to create a seal.

6. Lay the packets on a baking pan and bake for 15 minutes. Take it out of the oven and allow it to rest for 5 minutes. Be careful when opening the packet so that you don't get burned by steam. Garnish with cilantro and serve with rice.

Shrimp Skewers with Mango Salsa

Servings: 6

Macros Per Serving:

- ➢ 123 Calories
- ➢ 431 mg Sodium
- ➢ 11 g Protein
- ➢ 317 mg Potassium
- ➢ 213 mg Phosphorus

What You Need:

- ➢ For the Shrimp:
- ➢ Canola oil, 1 tsp
- ➢ Cleaned shrimp, tails on, 1 lb
- ➢ Minced ginger, 1-inch piece
- ➢ Honey, 2 tbsp
- ➢ Lime juice, 2 limes
- ➢ For the Salsa:
- ➢ Diced small red chili
- ➢ Diced sweet onion, .25 c
- ➢ Juice of a lime
- ➢ Diced and peeled mango
- ➢ Diced and seeded medium cucumber

What You Do:

1. For the shrimp: mix together the ginger, honey, and lime juice. Toss the shrimp to coat with the mixture.

2. Cover the shrimp and refrigerate them for a minimum of 30 minutes.

3. Thread the shrimp onto your skewers.

4. Heat up your grill to medium high and brush with some oil. Cook your skewers for 3 to 6 minutes on both sides. The shrimp should turn opaque when cooked through.

5. For the salsa: toss the lime juice, mango, cucumber, chili, and onion together in a small bowl. Once the shrimp is cooked, remove from skewers and add to salsa. Toss together and serve.

Desserts

Chocolate Beet Cake

Servings: 12

Macros Per Serving:

- 270 Calories
- 109 mg Sodium
- 6 g Protein
- 299 mg Potassium
- 111 mg Phosphorus

What You Need:

- Grated beets, 3 c
- Canola oil, .25 c
- Eggs, 4
- Unsweetened chocolate, 4 oz
- Phosphorus-free baking powder, 2 tsp
- All-purpose flour, 2 c
- Sugar, 1 c

What You Do:

1. Set your oven to 325° F. Grease 2 8-inch cake pans.
2. Mix the baking powder, flour, and sugar together. Set aside.
3. Chop up the chocolate as finely as you can and melt using a double boiler. A microwave can also be used, just don't let it burn. Allow the it to cool and mix into the oil and eggs.

4. Mix all of the wet ingredients into the flour mixture and combine everything together until well mixed.

5. Fold the beets in and pour the batter in the cake pans.

6. Let them bake for 40 to 50 minutes. To know it's done, the toothpick should come out clean when inserted to the cake. Remove in the oven and allow them to cool. Once cool, invert over a plate to remove.

7. This is great served with whipped cream and fresh berries.

Strawberry Pie

Servings: 8

Macros Per Serving:

➢ 265 Calories

➢ 143 mg Sodium

➢ 3 g Protein

➢ 183 mg Potassium

➢ 44 mg Phosphorus

What You Need:

➢ For the Crust:

➢ Graham cracker crumbs, 1.5 c

➢ Room-temperature unsalted butter, 5 tbsp

➢ Sugar, 2 tbsp

➢ For the Pie:

➢ Gelatin powder, 1.5 tsp

➢ Cornstarch, 3 tbsp

➢ Sugar, .75 c

➢ Sliced strawberries, 5 c, divided

➢ Water, 1 c

What You Do:

1. For the crust: heat your oven to 375° F. Grease a pie pan.
2. Combine the butter, crumbs, and sugar together and then press them into your pie pan.
3. Bake the crust for 10 to 15 minutes, until lightly browned. Take out of the oven and let it cool completely.

4. For the pie: crush up a cup of strawberries. Using a small pot, combine the sugar, water, gelatin, and cornstarch.

5. Bring the mixture in the pot up to a boil, lower the heat, and simmer until it has thickened.

6. Add in the crushed strawberries in the pot and let it simmer for another 5 minutes until the sauce has thickened up again. Set it off the heat and pour into a bowl. Cool until it comes to room temperature.

7. Toss the remaining berries with the sauce so that it is well distributed and pour into the pie crust and spread it out into an even layer.

8. Refrigerate the pie until cold. This will take about 3 hours.

Lemon Tart

Servings: 10

Macros Per Serving:

- 252 Calories
- 29 mg Sodium
- 4 g Protein
- 59 mg Potassium
- 55 mg Phosphorus

What You Need:

- For the Shell:
- All-purpose flour, 1.25 c
- Melted unsalted butter, 8 tbsp
- Sugar, 2tbsp
- For the Tart:
- Sugar, .5 c
- Eggs, 3
- Zest of a lemon
- Lemon juice, .5 c
- Powdered sugar
- Sliced lemon
- Butter, 4 tbsp

What You Do:

1. For the shell: combine the flour and sugar together and then drizzle in the melted butter. Mix everything together.

2. Add the flour mixture to your pan and use your hand to press the crust out on to the bottom and sides of the dish. Cover with plastic wrap and place the crust in the fridge for 30 minutes.

3. Place your oven to 350° F.

4. Prick the crust with a fork around 20 times and then bake it for 20 minutes. The crust should be golden. Allow the crust to cool completely before you add the filling.

5. For the tart: bring the lemon juice and zest to a boil in a medium pot. Set off the heat.

6. Combine the sugar and eggs together, and then slowly pour into the lemon juice, constantly whisking. Let this cook over medium heat, constantly stirring until it has thickened. Do this for around 6 to 8 minutes.

7. Add in the butter pieces and set off the heat. Stir until the butter has melted. Strain through a wire sieve into the tart crust. Refrigerate for 2 hours before you serve.

8. Top with powdered sugar and lemon slices.

Grape Skillet Galette

Servings: 6

Macros Per Serving:

- 172 Calories
- 65 mg Sodium
- 2 g Protein
- 69 mg Potassium
- 21 mg Phosphorus

What You Need:

- For the Crust:
- Unsweetened rice milk, .5 c
- Cold butter, 4 tbsp
- Sugar, 1 tbsp
- All-purpose flour, 1 c
- For the Galette:
- Cornstarch, 1 tbsp
- Sugar, .33 c
- Egg white
- Halved seedless grapes, 2 c

What You Do:

1. For the crust: add the sugar and the flour to a food processor and mix for a few seconds. Place in the butter and pulse until it looks like a coarse meal. Add in the rice milk and combine until the dough forms.

2. Place the dough on a clean surface and shape into a disc. Wrap it with a plastic wrap and place it in the fridge for 2 hours.

3. For the galette: set your oven to 425° F.

4. Mix the cornstarch and sugar and toss the grapes in.

5. Unwrap the dough and roll out on a floured surface. Press it into a 14-inch circle and place in a cast iron skillet.

6. Add the grape filling in the center and spread out to fill, leaving a 2-inch crust. Fold the edge over.

7. Brush the crust with egg white and cook for 20 to 25 minutes. The crust should be golden. Allow to rest for 20 minutes before you serve.

Berry Crumble

Servings: 12

Macros Per Serving:

- 167 Calories
- 3 mg Sodium
- 3 g Protein
- 155 mg Potassium
- 75 mg Phosphorus

What You Need:

- Melted unsalted butter, .25 c
- Cinnamon, 1 tsp
- Brown sugar, .25 c
- Rolled oats, .75 c
- All-purpose flour, .75 c
- Sugar, .25 c
- Frozen berries, 6 c

What You Do:

1. Set your oven to 375° F.
2. Toss the sugar and the berries together, then add to a medium casserole dish.
3. Mix together the cinnamon, brown sugar, oats, and flour. Pour in the melted butter and mix together.
4. Use your hands and press the crumble together into small pieces. Lay the clumps over the berries.
5. Bake for an hour. The top should be browned and crispy and berries should bubble. Let stand 30 minutes before serving.

Zesty Shortbread

Servings: 16

Macros Per Serving:

- ➢ 94 Calories
- ➢ 1 mg Sodium
- ➢ 1 g Protein
- ➢ 10 mg Potassium
- ➢ 10 mg Phosphorus

What You Need:

- ➢ Zest of a lemon
- ➢ Zest of a lime
- ➢ Unsalted butter, .5 c
- ➢ Powdered sugar, .5 c
- ➢ All-purpose flour, 1 c

What You Do:

1. Set your oven to 375° F.
2. Add both zests, butter, sugar, and flour to a food processor. Process until it forms a dough.
3. Measure out a tablespoon and roll into a ball. Place on a cookie sheet and continue to form the balls until the dough is used up.
4. Dip a cup in powdered sugar and press down the cookie dough to flatten.
5. Bake for 13 to 15 minutes. The edges should be browned. Place on a wire rack to cool. Keep in an airtight container for 5 days.

Grapefruit Sorbet

Servings: 6

Macros Per Serving:

- 109 Calories
- 2 mg Sodium
- 1 g Protein
- 318 mg Potassium
- 29 mg Phosphorus

What You Need:

- For the Simple Syrup:
- Thyme sprig
- Water, .25 c
- Sugar, .5 c
- For the Sorbet:
- Thyme simple syrup, .25 c
- Grapefruit juice, 6 pink grapefruit

What You Do:

1. For the simple syrup: add the thyme, water, and sugar to a small pot. Allow this to come to a boil and then turn off the heat. Refrigerate everything until cold. Strain to remove the thyme sprig.
2. Add a quarter cup of simple syrup and the grapefruit juice to a blender and process to combine.
3. Pour into an airtight container and freeze for 3 to 4 hours. It should be firm. Serve.

Tropical Granita

Servings: 4

Macros Per Serving:

- ➤ 103 Calories
- ➤ 3 mg Sodium
- ➤ 1 g Protein
- ➤ 145 mg Potassium
- ➤ 13 mg Phosphorus

What You Need:

- ➤ Fresh mint
- ➤ Juice of a lime
- ➤ Orange juice, 2 c
- ➤ Fresh or frozen mango chunks, .5 c
- ➤ Fresh or frozen pineapple chunks, 1 c

What You Do:

1. Mix the lime juice, orange juice, mango, and pineapple in a blender. Mix until smooth and add to a freezer-safe bowl. Freeze for 2 hours.
2. Use a fork and break the mixture up into smaller pieces. Serve with a garnish of mint leaves.

Drinks

Blueberry Burst

Servings: 2

Macros Per Serving:

- 131 Calories
- 60 mg Sodium
- 3 g Protein
- 146 mg Potassium
- 51 mg Phosphorus

What You Need:

- Ice cubes, 3
- Almond butter, 1 tbsp
- Unsweetened rice milk, 1 c
- Chopped collard greens, 1 c
- Blueberries, 1 c

What You Do:

1. Combine everything in a blender until smooth. Pour into 2 glasses and serve.

Apple and Cucumber Smoothie

Servings: 2

Macros Per Serving:

- ➢ 75 Calories
- ➢ 81 mg Sodium
- ➢ 1 g Protein
- ➢ 313 mg Potassium
- ➢ 34 mg Phosphorus

What You Need:

- ➢ Ice cubes, 3
- ➢ Spinach, 2 c
- ➢ Unsweetened rice milk, 1 c
- ➢ Chopped green apple, .5
- ➢ Chopped cucumber, .5

What You Do:

1. Place everything in a blender and mix until smooth. Pour into 2 glasses and serve.

Mint Papaya Water

Servings: 10

Macros Per Serving:

- 2 Calories
- 0 mg Sodium
- 0 g Protein
- 4 mg Potassium
- 0 mg Phosphorus

What You Need:

- Water, 10 c
- Chopped mint leaves, 2 tbsp
- Diced, seeded, peeled papaya, 1 c

What You Do:

1. Put all ingredients into a large pitcher. Place in the refrigerator to infuse overnight.

Peach Carrot Water

Servings: 10

Macros Per Serving:

- 3 Calories
- 0 mg Sodium
- 0 g Protein
- 4 mg Potassium
- 0 mg Phosphorus

What You Need:

- Water, 10 c
- Thyme sprigs, 3
- Lightly crushed peeled ginger, 1 inch
- Grated, peeled carrot, 1 large
- Chopped, pitted, peeled peaches, 2

What You Do:

1. Place all ingredients into a large pitcher. Give it a good stir. Place in the refrigerator to infuse overnight.

Cheesecake Mango Smoothie

Servings: 2

Macros Per Serving:

- 148 Calories
- 51 mg Sodium
- 2 g Protein
- 133 mg Potassium
- 54 mg Phosphorus

What You Need:

- Ice cubes, 3
- Ground nutmeg
- Split and scraped vanilla bean, .5
- Honey, 1 tsp
- Cream cheese, 2 tbsp
- Chopped, peeled mango, .5
- Unsweetened rice milk, 1 c

What You Do:

1. Process everything in a blender until smooth. Pour into 2 glasses to serve.

Melon Smoothie

Servings: 2

Macros Per Serving:

- 60 Calories
- 2 mg Sodium
- 1 g Protein
- 200 mg Potassium
- 27 mg Phosphorus

What You Need:

- Ice cubes, 3
- Lemon juice, 1 tbsp
- Chopped mint leaves, 1 tsp
- Strawberries, .5 c
- Watermelon cubes, 1 c

What You Do:

1. Mix everything in a blender until smooth. Pour into 2 glasses to serve.

Apple PieSmoothie

Servings: 2

Macros Per Serving:

- ➢ 95 Calories
- ➢ 8 mg Sodium
- ➢ 1 g Protein
- ➢ 200 mg Potassium
- ➢ 20 mg Phosphorus

What You Need:

- ➢ Ice cubes, 3
- ➢ Ground cloves
- ➢ Ground cinnamon, .5 tsp
- ➢ Vanilla, 1 tsp
- ➢ Water, 1 c
- ➢ Chopped spinach, .5 c
- ➢ Chopped, cored apples, 2

What You Do:

1. Mix everything in a blender until smooth and serve in 2 glasses.

Kiwi Smoothie

Servings: 2

Macros Per Serving:

➢ 101 Calories
➢ 11 mg Sodium
➢ 2 g Protein
➢ 200 mg Potassium
➢ 63 mg Phosphorus

What You Need:

➢ Ice cubes, 2
➢ Honey, 1 tsp
➢ Almonds, 2 tbsp
➢ Chopped kale, .5 c
➢ Chopped, peeled kiwi, 1
➢ Chopped avocado, .5
➢ Water, 1 c

What You Do:

1. Mix everything in a blender until smooth and serve in 2 glasses.

Pretty in Pink Smoothie

Servings: 2

Macros Per Serving:

- 137 Calories
- 50 mg Sodium
- 1 g Protein
- 197 mg Potassium
- 37 mg Phosphorus

What You Need:

- Ice cubes, 3
- Chopped cooked beet, .5 small
- Grated ginger, 1 tsp
- Flaxseed, 2 tsp
- Unsweetened rice milk, 1 c
- Chopped orange, .5
- Chopped pear, 1

What You Do:

1. Mix everything in a blender until smooth and serve in 2 glasses.

Cucumber Raspberry Smoothie

Servings: 2

Macros Per Serving:

➢ 107 Calories

➢ 42 mg Sodium

➢ 5 g Protein

➢ 135 mg Potassium

➢ 37 mg Phosphorus

What You Need:

➢ Ice cubes, 3

➢ Honey, 1 tsp

➢ Chia seeds, 2 tsp

➢ Unsweetened rice milk, 1 c

➢ Diced English cucumber, .5

➢ Raspberries, 1 c

What You Do:

1. Mix everything in a blender until smooth and serve in 2 glasses.

Blackberry Surprise Smoothie

Servings: 2

Macros Per Serving:

➢ 118 Calories

➢ 55 mg Sodium

➢ 2 g Protein

➢ 193 mg Potassium

➢ 25 mg Phosphorus

What You Need:

➢ Ice cubes, 3

➢ Ground cinnamon, .25 tsp

➢ Honey, .5 tsp

➢ Vanilla, .5 tsp

➢ Unsweetened rice milk, 1 c

➢ Chopped kale, .5 c

➢ Blackberries, 1 c

What You Do:

1. Mix everything in a blender until smooth and serve in 2 glasses.

Strawberry Cheesecake Smoothie

Servings: 2

Macros Per Serving:

- 114 Calories
- 102 mg Sodium
- 1 g Protein
- 132 mg Potassium
- 33 mg Phosphorus

What You Need:

- Ice cubes, 3-5
- Vanilla, 1 tsp
- Honey, .5 tsp
- Room temperature cream cheese, 2 tbsp
- Hulled strawberries, 1 c
- Unsweetened rice milk, 1 c

What You Do:

1. Add everything to a blender and mix until smooth. Pour into 2 glasses and serve.

Watermelon Kiwi Smoothie

Servings: 2

Macros Per Serving:

- 67 Calories
- 3 mg Sodium
- 1 g Protein
- 278 mg Potassium
- 28 mg Phosphorus

What You Need:

- Ice, 1 c
- Peeled kiwifruit
- Watermelon chunks, 2 c

What You Do:

1. Add everything to a blender and mix until smooth. Divide into 2 glasses and serve.

Vanilla Chia Smoothie

Servings: 2

Macros Per Serving:

- ➢ 143 Calories
- ➢ 73 mg Sodium
- ➢ 3 g Protein
- ➢ 93 mg Potassium
- ➢ 3 mgPhosphorus

What You Need:

- ➢ Ground cloves, .25 tsp
- ➢ Ground cardamom, .25 tsp
- ➢ Ground ginger, .5 tsp
- ➢ Ground cinnamon, .5 tsp
- ➢ Chia seeds, 2 tbsp
- ➢ Honey, 1 tsp
- ➢ Ice, 1 c
- ➢ Vanilla, 1 tsp
- ➢ Black tea bags, 2
- ➢ Unsweetened rice milk, 1 c

What You Do:

2. Add the milk to a pot and heat to just steaming. Place the tea bags into the milk and steep for 5 minutes. Discard tea bags.
3. Place everything into your blender and mix until smooth. Pour into 2 glasses and serve.

Mint Lassi

Servings: 2

Macros Per Serving:

- ➢ 114 Calories
- ➢ 43 mg Sodium
- ➢ 10 g Protein
- ➢ 179 mg Potassium
- ➢ 158 mg Phosphorus

What You Need:

- ➢ Water, .5 c
- ➢ Unsweetened yogurt, 1 c
- ➢ Mint leaves, .5 c
- ➢ Cumin seeds, 1 tsp

What You Do:

1. Toast the cumin in a dry skillet until fragrant, about 1 to 2 minutes.
2. Add to a blender, along with the other ingredients, and process until smooth.
3. Divide into 2 glasses and serve.

Fennel Digestive Cooler

Servings: 2

Macros Per Serving:

- ➢ 163 Calories
- ➢ 141 mg Sodium
- ➢ 3 g Protein
- ➢ 205 mg Potassium
- ➢ 57 mg Phosphorus

What You Need:

- ➢ Honey, 1 tbsp
- ➢ Ground cloves, .25 tsp
- ➢ Ground fennel seeds, .25 c
- ➢ Unsweetened rice milk, 2 c

What You Do:

1. Blend everything in a blender and allow to rest for 30 minutes.
2. Pour through a wire sieve lined with cheesecloth. Pour into 2 glasses and serve.

Berry Mint Water

Servings: 8

Macros Per Serving:

- 7 Calories
- 0 mg Sodium
- 0 g Protein
- 28 mg Potassium
- 4 mg Phosphorus

What You Need:

- Mint springs, 3
- Blackberries, .5 c
- Strawberries, .5 c
- Water, 8 c

What You Do:

1. Mix everything in a glass pitcher and allow to chill for an hour before serving.

Winter Berry Milkshake

Servings: 4

Macros Per Serving:

- 45 Calories
- 29 mg Sodium
- 2 g Protein
- 118 mg Potassium
- 33 mg Phosphorus

What You Need:

- Ice cubes, 3
- Blackberries, .5 c
- Blueberries, .5 c
- Unsweetened rice milk, 1 c

What You Do:

1. Add everything to a blender and mix until smooth. Serve in 4 glasses.

Apple Banana Smoothie

Servings: 4

Macros Per Serving:

- 182 Calories
- 14 mg Sodium
- 2 g Protein
- 300 mg Potassium
- 70 mg Phosphorus

What You Need:

- Low-fat coconut milk, 1 c
- Stevia, 1 tbsp
- Filtered water, 2 c
- Peeled and cored apple
- Banana

What You Do:

1. Mix everything in a blender until smooth and serve in 4 glasses over ice.

Anti-Inflammatory Smoothie

Servings: 4

Macros Per Serving:

- ➢ 48 Calories
- ➢ 6 mg Sodium
- ➢ 1 g Protein
- ➢ 203 mg Potassium
- ➢ 17 mg Phosphorus

What You Need:

- ➢ Sprig of mint
- ➢ Water, .5 c
- ➢ Ice cubes, .5 c
- ➢ Chopped cabbage, 1 c
- ➢ Frozen peaches, 1 c
- ➢ White grapes, 1 c

What You Do:

1. Mix everything in a blender until smooth. Serve in 4 glasses with a sprig of mint.

Tropical Juice

Servings: 2

Macros Per Serving:

- 55 Calories
- 111 mg Sodium
- 7 g Protein
- 129 mg Potassium
- 11 mg Phosphorus

What You Need:

- Water, 1 c
- Low-fat coconut milk, .5 c
- Chunked pineapple, 2 c

What You Do:

1. Blend all of the ingredients together until smooth. Serve in 2 glasses.

Lemon Smoothie

Servings: 2

Macros Per Serving:

- ➢ 49 Calories
- ➢ 110 mg Sodium
- ➢ 8 g Protein
- ➢ 112 mg Potassium
- ➢ 10 mg Phosphorus

What You Need:

- ➢ Brown sugar, 2 tbsp
- ➢ Liquid egg whites, 4
- ➢ Lemon juice, 2 tbsp

What You Do:

1. Blend everything together and serve in 2 glasses. Garnish with lemon.

Blueberry Smoothie

Servings: 4

Macros Per Serving:

- 108 Calories
- 27 mg Sodium
- 9 g Protein
- 183 mg Potassium
- 42 mg Phosphorus

What You Need:

- Sugar-free apple juice, 14 oz
- Ice cubes, 8
- Protein powder, 6 tbsp
- Splenda, 8 packs
- Frozen blueberries, 1 c

What You Do:

1. Add everything to a blender and mix. Serve in 4 glasses.

Pineapple Smoothie

Servings: 1

Macros Per Serving:

- 268 Calories
- 93 mg Sodium
- 18 g Protein
- 237 mg Potassium
- 160 mg Phosphorus

What You Need:

- Ice cubes, 2
- Water, .5 c
- Vanilla protein powder, 1 scoop
- Pineapple sorbet, .75 c

What You Do:

1. Mix everything in the blender and enjoy.

Fruity Smoothie

Servings: 2

Macros Per Serving:

- ➢ 186 Calories
- ➢ 62 mg Sodium
- ➢ 23 g Protein
- ➢ 282 mg Potassium
- ➢ 118 mg Phosphorus

What You Need:

- ➢ Crushed ice, 1 c
- ➢ Cold water, 1 c
- ➢ Vanilla protein powder, 2 scoops
- ➢ Canned fruit cocktail, 8 oz, with juice

What You Do:

1. Mix everything together in a blender and serve in 2 glasses.

Ginger Green Tea

Servings: 2

Macros Per Serving:

- ➤ 20 Calories
- ➤ 4 mg Sodium
- ➤ 1 g Protein
- ➤ 106 mg Potassium
- ➤ 9 mg Phosphorus

What You Need:

- ➤ Crystallized ginger, .25 c
- ➤ Lemon
- ➤ Hot green tea, 2 c

What You Do:

1. Mix the tea and the ginger together and chill for 3 hours.
2. Strain and serve in 2 glasses garnished with a wedge of lemon.

Strawberry Smoothie

Servings: 2

Macros Per Serving:

- ➢ 80 Calories
- ➢ 58 mg Sodium
- ➢ 4 g Protein
- ➢ 276 mg Potassium
- ➢ 73 mg Phosphorus

What You Need:

- ➢ Unsweetened rice milk, 1 c
- ➢ Sliced strawberries, 1 c

What You Do:

1. Blend everything together and serve in 2 glasses over ice.

Vegetable Main Dishes

Creamy Pesto Pasta

Servings: 4

Macros Per Serving:

- 394 Calories
- 4 mg Sodium
- 10 g Protein
- 148 mg Potassium
- 54 mg Phosphorus

What You Need:

- Pepper
- EVOO, 25 c
- Garlic, 3 cloves
- Walnut pieces, .33 c
- Packed arugula, 2 c
- Packed basil, 2 c
- Linguine noodles, 8 oz

What You Do:

1. Fill a pot halfway full with water and allow to boil. Cook the noodles until they reach al dente. Drain.
2. Place the garlic, walnuts, arugula, and basil to a food processor and mix until coarsely ground. While the processor is on, slowly add in the oil and mix until creamy. Add in some pepper.
3. Toss the noodles with the pesto and enjoy.

Tofu and Rice Bowls

Servings: 4

Macros Per Serving:

➢ 393 Calories

➢ 54 mg Sodium

➢ 12 g Protein

➢ 362 mg Potassium

➢ 211 mg Phosphorus

What You Need:

➢ For the Dressing:

➢ Water, .25 c

➢ Tahini, 1 tbsp

➢ EVOO, 2 tbsp

➢ Minced garlic, 2 cloves

➢ Apple cider vinegar, 2 tbsp

➢ For the Salad:

➢ Extra-firm tofu, 14 oz

➢ Sunflower seeds, .25 c

➢ Grated carrot, 2

➢ Grated and peeled beet

➢ Mixed salad greens, 4 c

➢ White rice, 1 c

➢ Sesame oil, 1 tbsp

What You Do:

1. Mix the dressing ingredients together and place to the side.

2. Set your oven to 350° F. Line the baking sheet with parchment paper.

3. Slice the tofu into half-inch thick rectangles. Toss in sesame oil and lay it out on the prepared baking sheet. Bake for 15 minutes.

4. Cook the rice according to directions.

5. Place a scoop of rice in 4 bowls and top each with a cup of salad greens and equal amounts of sunflower seeds, carrots, and beets. Top with the tofu and some dressing.

Vegetable Barley

Servings: 6

Macros Per Serving:

- ➤ 156 Calories
- ➤ 16 mg Sodium
- ➤ 4 g Protein
- ➤ 220 mg Potassium
- ➤ 83 mg Phosphorus

What You Need:

- ➤ Minced parsley, 1 tbsp
- ➤ Water, 2 c
- ➤ White rice, .5 c
- ➤ Barley, .5 c
- ➤ Sliced carrot, 1
- ➤ Diced red bell pepper, 1
- ➤ Cauliflower florets, 2 c
- ➤ Minced garlic, 2 tsp
- ➤ Chopped sweet onion, 1 medium
- ➤ Olive oil, 1 tbsp

What You Do:

1. Warm the oil in a large skillet. Add in the onion and garlic. Cook until soft.

2. Put the carrot, bell pepper, and cauliflower into the skillet and cook for another 5 minutes. Add in the water, rice, and barley and allow to boil.

3. Place lid on skillet. Turn heat down and simmer for 25 minutes. All the liquid needs to be absorbed. The rice and barley should be tender. Sprinkle with parsley.

Mushroom Noodles

Servings: 4

Macros Per Serving:

- 163 Calories
- 199 mg Sodium
- 2 g Protein
- 200 mg Potassium
- 69 mg Phosphorus

What You Need:

- Low-sodium soy sauce, 1 tbsp
- Sliced scallions, 2
- Sliced red bell pepper, 1
- Julienned carrot, 1
- Sliced yellow bell pepper, 1
- Minced garlic, 2 tsp
- Sliced mushrooms, 2 c
- Sesame oil, 2 tsp
- Rice noodles, 4 c

What You Do:

1. Cook the rice noodles as stated on the package. Set these to the side.
2. Warm the oil in a skillet. Place the garlic and mushrooms and sauté for 7 minutes until caramelized.
3. Add in the scallions, carrot, and bell peppers and cook for another 5 minutes.
4. Add in the rice noodles and soy sauce. Give everything a good toss to coat the noodles, then serve.

Fried Rice

Servings: 6

Macros Per Serving:

➢ 204 Calories
➢ 223 mg Sodium
➢ 8 g Protein
➢ 147 mg Potassium
➢ 120 mg Phosphorus

What You Need:

➢ Eggs, 4
➢ Low-sodium soy sauce, 1 tbsp
➢ Cooked rice, 4 c
➢ Grated ginger, 1 tbsp
➢ Chopped cilantro, 2 tbsp
➢ Chopped scallion, 1
➢ Chopped carrots, 1 c
➢ Minced garlic, 1 tsp
➢ Olive oil, 1 tbsp

What You Do:

1. Warm the oil in a large skillet. Put in the garlic and ginger and cook for 3 minutes. Add the cilantro, scallion, and carrots and cook for another 5 minutes.
2. Add in the soy sauce and rice and cook for another 5 minutes just until rice is warmed through. Scoop the rice over to one side and put the eggs in the empty spot.
3. Scramble the eggs and mix everything together.

Cauliflower Cakes

Servings: 6

Macros Per Serving:

- ➢ 141 Calories
- ➢ 82 mg Sodium
- ➢ 7 g Protein
- ➢ 178 mg Potassium
- ➢ 119 mg Phosphorus

What You Need:

- ➢ Pepper
- ➢ Ground nutmeg, .25 tsp
- ➢ Shredded cheddar cheese, .5 c
- ➢ Eggs, 2
- ➢ Plain yogurt, .25 c
- ➢ Cooked rice, 2 c
- ➢ Chopped cauliflower, 2 c

What You Do:

1. Warm your oven to 350° F. Lightly brush with olive oil the 6 cups in a normal muffin pan.
2. Blanch the cauliflower and drain well.
3. Place the cauliflower into a large bowl along with nutmeg, cheese, eggs, yogurt, and rice. Sprinkle with pepper. Stir well to incorporate all the ingredients.
4. Divide this mixture evenly in the 6 muffin cups. Allow this to bake for 20 minutes. Everything should be golden.
5. Remove from the oven and let cool for 5 minutes. Loosen the edges with a knife to remove easily.

Veggie Burgers

Servings: 4

Macros Per Serving:

- ➢ 247 Calories
- ➢ 36 mg Sodium
- ➢ 8 g Protein
- ➢ 183 mg Potassium
- ➢ 120 mg Phosphorus

What You Need:

- ➢ Olive oil, 1 tbsp
- ➢ Zest and juice of one lime
- ➢ Chopped basil, 2 tsp
- ➢ Minced garlic, 1 tsp
- ➢ Chopped parsley, 2 tbsp
- ➢ Eggs, 2
- ➢ Cooked lentil, rinsed and drained, .5 c
- ➢ Cooked white rice, 2.5 c

What You Do:

1. Place the garlic, lime zest, lime juice, basil, parsley, eggs, lentils, and rice into a food processor and pulse until mixture sticks together.
2. Place this mixture into a bowl and place in the refrigerator for an hour.
3. Form the mixture into 4 patties.
4. Warm the oil in a large skillet. Place in the patties and cook until they have browned on the bottom for around 5 minutes. Turn patties over and cook for another 5 minutes.
5. Serve hot with topping of choice.

Spinach Falafel Wrap

Servings: 4

Macros Per Serving:

- 241 Calories
- 285 mg Sodium
- 8 g Protein
- 245 mg Potassium
- 110 mg Phosphorus

What You Need:

- Tortillas, 4
- Pepper
- Juice of a lemon
- Minced garlic, 2 cloves
- Unsweetened yogurt, .25 c
- Canola oil, 2 tbsp, divided
- Flour, .75 c
- Ground cumin, 2 tsp
- Drained and rinsed chickpeas, 15 oz
- Baby spinach, 6 oz
- Salad greens
- Red onion, 2 slices
- Cucumber cut in spears

What You Do:

1. Lay the spinach in a mesh sieve and pour boiling water over to wilt. Let it cool and remove as much water as you can.

2. Blend the flour, cumin, chickpeas, and spinach together in a food processor.
3. Press the mixture into tablespoon-size balls and flatten into patties.
4. Pour a tablespoon of oil to a pan and add in the falafels, cooking 2 to 3 minutes on each side. Repeat until all falafels are cooked.
5. Mix the pepper, lemon juice, garlic, and yogurt together.
6. Place 3 falafels on a tortilla with a couple of cucumber spears, onion rings, and salad greens.
7. Top with a tablespoon of the sauce and serve.

Stir Fried Bean Sprouts and Broccoli

Servings: 2

Macros Per Serving:

- 97 Calories
- 55 mg Sodium
- 2 g Protein
- 63 mg Potassium
- 262 mg Phosphorus

What You Need:

- Rice wine vinegar, 1 tbsp
- Chinese five spice, 1 tsp
- Minced garlic, 2 cloves
- Coconut oil, 1 tbsp
- Minced ginger, 1-inch piece
- Bean sprouts, .25 c
- Sprouting broccoli, 1 c

What You Do:

1. Add the oil to a wok or skillet and heat to high. Add the ginger, garlic, and spices, cooking for a minute.
2. Mix in the veggies and vinegar. Sauté for 8 to 10 minutes.
3. Serve over rice.

Green Bean Pesto Pasta

Servings: 4

Macros Per Serving:

- 262 Calories
- 5 mg Sodium
- 6 g Protein
- 183 mg Potassium
- 68 mg Phosphorus

What You Need:

- Pepper, 1 tsp
- Trimmed green beans, 2 c
- Juiced lemon
- Wild garlic leaves, .25 c
- EVOO, .25 c
- Washed spinach, .5 c
- Washed basil, .5 c
- White penne pasta, 2 c

What You Do:

1. Bring water to a boil and allow the pasta to cook for 15 to 20 minutes.

2. Meanwhile, blend everything, except for the beans, until it reaches your desired consistency.

3. Steam the green beans over the pot of pasta during the last 10 minutes.

4. Drain the pasta and toss together with the green beans and the pesto. Sprinkle on some pepper.

Soups and Salads

Creamy Broccoli Soup

Servings: 4

Macros Per Serving:

- 88 Calories
- 281 mg Sodium
- 4 g Protein
- 201 mg Potassium
- 87 mg Phosphorus

What You Need:

- Parmesan, .25 c
- Unsweetened rice milk, 1 c
- Pepper
- Low-sodium vegetable broth, 4 c
- Chopped broccoli, 2 c
- Chopped onion, .5
- EVOO, 1 tsp

What You Do:

1. Heat the oil in a medium pot over medium-high heat.
2. Cook the onions until they become soft. Mix in the broth and broccoli and season with pepper.
3. Let it come to a boil, then turn the heat down. Simmer uncovered for 10 minutes. The broccoli should be tender.
4. Pour into a blender and carefully mix until smooth. Add back to the pot and mix with the parmesan. Enjoy.

Brie and Beetroot Salad

Servings: 2

Macros Per Serving:

- 212 Calories
- 137 mg Sodium
- 4 g Protein
- 236 mg Potassium
- 51 mg Phosphorus

What You Need:

- Pepper, 1 tsp
- Brie, 1 oz
- Canned diced beets, .5 c
- Romaine lettuce, 1 c
- Chopped dill, 1 tbsp
- Dijon mustard, 1 tsp
- Juice of an orange
- EVOO, 2 tbsp

What You Do:

Combine the dill, mustard, orange juice, and oil in a salad bowl.

Place the lettuce in dressing and toss together.

Serve topped with the brie and beetroot. Season with pepper.

Vegetable Minestrone

Servings: 6

Macros Per Serving:

- 100 Calories
- 7 mg Sodium
- 4 g Protein
- 200 mg Potassium
- 70 mg Phosphorus

What You Need:

- Parmesan cheese, 1 ounce
- Pepper
- Shredded kale, .5 c
- Diced zucchini, 1
- Chopped tomatoes, 2 medium
- Sodium-free chicken stock, 2 c
- Minced garlic, 1 tsp
- Diced celery, 1 stalk
- Chopped onion, .5 sweet
- Olive oil, 1 tsp

What You Do:

1. Warm the oil in a large pot.
2. Put the garlic, celery, and onion into the pot and cook for 5 minutes until soft.
3. Add in the zucchini, tomatoes, and stock. Stir well and allow to boil. Turn heat down and simmer 15 minutes.
4. Add in kale, sprinkle in some pepper. Stir well. Sprinkle with parmesan cheese.

Cabbage Soup

Servings: 8

Macros Per Serving:

- 62 Calories
- 61 mg Sodium
- 2 g Protein
- 200 mg Potassium
- 32 mg Phosphorus

What You Need:

- Chopped thyme, 2 tbsp
- Pepper
- Diced tomatoes, 2
- Diced carrots, 2
- Shredded cabbage, .5 head
- Sodium-free chicken stock, 1 c
- Water, 6 c
- Minced garlic, 2 tsp
- Chopped onion, .5
- Olive oil, 1 tbsp

What You Do:

1. Warm the oil in a large saucepan.
2. Add in the onion and garlic, cooking until they become soft.
3. Add in tomatoes, carrots, cabbage, chicken stock, and water. Stir well and let everything come to a boil
4. Turn the heat down and let everything simmer until the veggies become tender, about 30 minutes.
5. Sprinkle with black pepper. Stir well and enjoy.

Mushroom "Miso" Soup

Servings: 6

Macros Per Serving:

- 56 Calories
- 118 mg Sodium
- 2 g Protein
- 198 mg Potassium
- 43 mgPhosphorus

What You Need:

- Chopped scallions, 2
- Grated carrot, .5 c
- Rice vinegar, .25 c
- Julienned snow peas, 1 c
- Grated ginger, 1 tbsp
- Low-sodium soy sauce, 1 tsp
- Dried mushroom, 2 ounces
- Water, 6 c

What You Do:

1. Pour 2 cups water into a small pan. Place on high heat and allow the water to boil.

2. Put the dried mushroom into a bowl and cover them with boiling water. Let this sit for 30 minutes. Take out of water and slice.

3. Put the ginger, soy sauce, vinegar, 4 cups of water, and mushroom water into a large pot. Allow this to come to a boil.

4. Put in the carrots, snow peas, and mushrooms. Lower the heat to simmer and cook 5 minutes. Ladle into bowls and top with scallions.

Carrot Soup

Servings: 4

Macros Per Serving:

- 113 Calories
- 30 mg Sodium
- 1 g Protein
- 200 mg Potassium
- 50 mg Phosphorus

What You Need:

- Chopped cilantro, 1 tbsp
- Coconut milk, .5 c
- Grated ginger, 2 tsp
- Ground turmeric, 1 tsp
- Chopped carrots, 3
- Water, 4 c
- Minced garlic, 1 tsp
- Chopped onion, .5
- Olive oil, 1 tbsp

What You Do:

1. Warm the oil in a large pot. Cook the garlic, ginger, and onion for 3 minutes.
2. Mix in turmeric, carrots, and water. Allow to boil, then turn the heat down to a simmer for 20 minutes until carrots are soft.

3. Put the soup into a blender and process with coconut milk until smooth. Be careful with hot liquids in a blender as it can get violent. Always put a kitchen towel over the top and hold on.
4. Put the blended soup back into the pan and warm back up.
5. Ladle into bowls and sprinkle some cilantro.

Cucumber Watermelon Salad

Servings: 6

Macros Per Serving:

- 42 Calories
- 3 mg Sodium
- 1 g Protein
- 200 mg Potassium
- 27 mg Phosphorus

What You Need:

- Chopped cilantro, 1 tbsp
- Lemon juice, 2 tbsp
- Chopped scallion, 1
- Cherry tomatoes, 1 c
- Diced English cucumber, 1
- Diced watermelon, 3 c

What You Do:

1. Toss all of the ingredients together in a large bowl.
2. Chill for 30 minutes, then serve.

Berry Salad

Macros Per Serving:

- ➢ 82 Calories
- ➢ 87 mg Sodium
- ➢ 3 g Protein
- ➢ 200 mg Potassium
- ➢ 63 mg Phosphorus

What You Need:

- ➢ Chopped basil, 2 tbsp
- ➢ Chopped pistachios, 2 tbsp
- ➢ Strawberries, 1 c
- ➢ Diced tomatoes, 1
- ➢ Blueberries, 1 c
- ➢ Raspberries, 1 c
- ➢ Shredded lettuce, 4 c

What You Do:

1. Divide the tomatoes, berries, and lettuce into 4 plates, as well as the basil and pistachios.
2. Serve and enjoy.

Beet and Carrot Soup

Servings: 4

Macros per Serving:

- ➢ 112 Calories
- ➢ 129 mg Sodium
- ➢ 3 g Protein
- ➢ 468 mg Potassium
- ➢ 57 mg Phosphorus

What You Need:

- ➢ Yogurt
- ➢ Pepper
- ➢ Unsweetened rice milk, 3 c
- ➢ Curry powder, 1 tbsp
- ➢ Chopped carrot, 5
- ➢ Large red beet

What You Do:

1. Set the oven to 400° F.
2. Wrap the beet in foil and bake for 45 minutes. You should be able to easily pierce it with a fork. Allow the beat to cool.
3. Add the carrots to a pot and cover with water. Let it come up to a boil, then turn the heat down. Place on a lid and let it cook for 10 minutes. The carrots should be tender.
4. Add the carrots and beet to a food processor and mix them together until they become smooth.
5. Mix in the milk and curry powder. Sprinkle in some pepper.
6. Serve with some yogurt on top.

Celery-Arugula Salad

Servings: 4

Macros Per Serving:

- 45 Calories
- 47 mg Sodium
- 1 g Protein
- 47 mg Potassium
- 23 mg Phosphorus

What You Need:

- Parmesan, 2 tbsp
- Pepper
- White wine vinegar, 2 tbsp
- EVOO, 1 tbsp
- Packed arugula, 2 c
- Diced celery stalks, 3
- Sliced shallot

What You Do:

1. Mix the oil, vinegar, and pepper together.
2. Combine all of the remaining ingredients, except the parmesan, in a bowl and toss together.
3. Drizzle the salad with the dressing and serve with some parmesan cheese.

Red Coleslaw with Apple

Servings: 4

Macros Per Serving:

- 94 Calories
- 281 mg Sodium
- 2 g Protein
- 303 mg Potassium
- 28 mg Phosphorus

What You Need:

- Pepper
- Diced tart apple
- Lemon juice, 2 lemons
- EVOO, 1 tbsp
- Honey, 1 tbsp
- Chopped scallions, .25 c
- Shredded carrots, .5 c
- Shredded cabbage, 3 c

What You Do:

1. Add everything to a bowl and mix together.
2. Chill the salad for 30 minutes.
3. Sprinkle on some pepper and serve.

Watercress and Pear Salad

Servings: 4

Macros Per Serving:

- 144 Calories
- 134 mg Sodium
- 3 g Protein
- 310 mg Potassium
- 70 mg Phosphorus

What You Need:

- Crumbled feta, 1 oz
- Cored pear cut into wedges, 2
- EVOO, 2 tbsp
- Washed bunch of watercress
- Honey, 1 tsp
- White wine vinegar, 1 tbsp
- Dijon mustard, 1 tsp
- Chopped onion, .25 c

What You Do:

Blend the honey, vinegar, olive oil, mustard, and onion together until smooth.

1. Toss the watercress in the dressing and place on 4 plates.
2. Top with the pear slices and feta.

Mixed Greens and Citrus Salad

Servings: 4

Macros Per Serving:

- 142 Calories
- 137 mg Sodium
- 3 g Protein
- 219 mg Potassium
- 116 mg Phosphorus

What You Need:

- Dried cranberries, 4 tbsp
- Sliced peeled lemon, .5
- Sliced peeled orange
- Pepper
- EVOO, 2 tsp
- Juice of a lemon
- Pepitas, .25 c
- Mixed salad greens, 4 c
- Kalamata olives, 4 tbsp

What You Do:

1. Toss the olive oil, lemon juice, pepitas, and greens together. Season with pepper.
2. Place on 4 plates and top with a few slices of lemon and orange.
3. Serve topped with a tablespoon of cranberries and olives per plate.

Watercress and Citrus

Servings: 2

Macros Per Serving:

- 304 Calories
- 33 mg Sodium
- 2 g Protein
- 392 mg Potassium
- 57 mg Phosphorus

What You Need:

- Sliced orange
- Watercress, 1 c
- Pepper
- Grated ginger, 2 tsp
- Cranberries, .5 c
- EVOO, 4 tsp
- Balsamic vinegar, 2 tbsp

What You Do:

1. Mix the oil and vinegar together and stir in the pepper, ginger, and cranberries.
2. Add the orange and watercress, and toss to coat.
3. Allow it to chill for 15 minutes before serving.

Strawberry Mint Salad

Servings: 2

Macros Per Serving:

- ➢ 26 Calories
- ➢ 2 mg Sodium
- ➢ 1 g Protein
- ➢ 118 mg Potassium
- ➢ 18 mg Phosphorus

What You Need:

- ➢ Balsamic vinegar, 1 tsp
- ➢ Chopped mint, 1 tbsp
- ➢ Sliced strawberries

What You Do:

1. Toss all of the ingredients together and serve.

Zesty Spinach Salad

Macros Per Serving:

- 73 Calories
- 35 mg Sodium
- 2 g Protein
- 353 mg Potassium
- 33 mg Phosphorus

What You Need:

- Peeled mandarin oranges, 2
- Baby spinach, 6 oz
- Pepper
- EVOO, 1 tbsp
- Juice and zest of mandarin orange

What You Do:

2. Whisk together the pepper, olive oil, orange juice, and the orange zest.
3. Toss the orange pieces and spinach together, then drizzle with the dressing.
4. Toss together, then serve.

Pepper Soup

Servings: 4

Macros Per Serving:

- 152 Calories
- 58 mg Sodium
- 5 g Protein
- 400 mg Potassium
- 92 mg Phosphorus

What You Need:

- Chicken stock, 3 c
- Chopped habanero, 2
- Chopped garlic, 2 cloves
- Chopped red bell pepper, 4
- Chopped red onion
- EVOO, 2.5 tbsp

What You Do:

1. Place the oil, peppers, and onions to a skillet and cook for 5 minutes.
2. Add in the habanero and the garlic. Cooking for 3 to 4 minutes.
3. Add in the stock and let it come to a boil. Turn the heat down and allow to simmer for 30 minutes.
4. Cool the soup slightly, and then add to a blender, mixing until smooth.
5. Sprinkle with pepper. Serve.

Radish and Cucumber Salad

Servings: 6

Macros Per Serving:

- 69 Calories
- 29 mg Sodium
- 2 g Protein
- 386 mg Potassium
- 52 mg Phosphorus

What You Need:

- Pepper
- EVOO, 1 tbsp
- Apple cider vinegar, .25 c
- Sliced onion, .5
- Sliced radishes, 1 bunch
- Sliced cucumber, 2 large

What You Do:

1. Toss the vegetables together.
2. Add in the olive oil and vinegar and toss together.
3. Season with some pepper and serve.

Apple and Watercress Salad

Servings: 2

Macros Per Serving:

- ➤ 80 Calories
- ➤ 121 mg Sodium
- ➤ 4 g Protein
- ➤ 120 mg Potassium
- ➤ 48 mg Phosphorus

What You Need:

- ➤ Diced apple, .5
- ➤ Watercress, 1 c
- ➤ White wine vinegar, 1 tsp

What You Do:

1. Toss all ingredients together and enjoy.

Snacks and Sides

Cinnamon Apple Chips

Servings: 4

Macros Per Serving:

➢ 96 Calories

➢ 2 mg Sodium

➢ 1 g Protein

➢ 198 mg Potassium

➢ 0 mg Phosphorus

What You Need:

➢ Ground cinnamon, 1 tsp

➢ Apples, 4

What You Do:

1. Set your oven to 350° F. Line a baking sheet with parchment.
2. Core your apples and slice them into 1/8-inch thick slices.
3. Toss the apple slices in the cinnamon. Spread the apple out onto the baking sheet in a single layer.
4. Cook them for 2 to 3 hours, or until the apples are dry.
5. While they are hot, they will still be soft. They will crisp up as they cool.
6. Keep them stored in an airtight container. They will last this way for about 4 days.

Walnut Pilaf

Servings: 4

Macros Per Serving:

- 233 Calories
- 88 mg Sodium
- 6 g Protein
- 179 mg Potassium
- 104 mg Phosphorus

What You Need:

- Chopped toasted walnuts, 1 tbsp
- Low-sodium chicken stock, 2 c
- Basmati rice, 1 c
- Chopped sweet onion, 1/4
- Chopped parsley, 2 tbsp
- Walnut oil, 1 tsp

What You Do:

1. Warm the oil in a pan and mix in the rice and onion. Allow this to cook for 5 minutes, stirring constantly. Set it off the heat.
2. Add in chicken stock, turn the heat up to bring it to a boil. Once boiling, put a lid on it, turn the heat back down so that it simmers for about 25 minutes.
3. The liquid should be completely absorbed. Add in the parsley and walnuts. Stir well.
4. Serve and enjoy.

German Cabbage

Servings: 4

Macros Per Serving:

- 62 Calories
- 14 mg Sodium
- 1 g Protein
- 161 mg Potassium
- 23 mg Phosphorus

What You Need:

- Dry mustard, .5 tsp
- Apple cider vinegar, 3 tbsp
- Caraway seed, .5 tsp
- Sugar, 1 tbsp
- Chopped sweet onion, .25 large
- Chopped, cored, and peeled pear. 1
- Shredded red cabbage, 5 c
- Olive oil, 1 tbsp

What You Do:

1. Warm the oil in a pan.
2. Put the onion, pear, and cabbage in the pan and sauté for about 10 minutes until cabbage is tender.
3. In a small bowl, add mustard, caraway seed, sugar, and vinegar. Stir to mix well.
4. Pour into pan with cabbage and stir well. Cover the pan and reduce the heat. Simmer for about 5 minutes.
5. Serve and enjoy.

Butternut Squash

Servings: 8

Macros Per Serving:

- 45 Calories
- 5 mg Sodium
- 1 g Protein
- 200 mg Potassium
- 19 mg Phosphorus

What You Need:

- Pepper
- Chopped fresh thyme, 1 tsp
- Chopped sweet onion, .5 medium
- Peeled, seeded, and cubed butternut squash, 4 c
- Olive oil, 1 tbsp

What You Do:

1. Warm the oil a large skillet.
2. Cook the butternut squash in the pan for about 15 minutes. Squash needs to be fork tender.
3. Add thyme and onion and cook for another 5 minutes.
4. Sprinkle with pepper.
5. Serve and enjoy.

Herbed Cauliflower

Servings: 4

Macros Per Serving:

➢ 82 Calories

➢ 122 mg Sodium

➢ 1 g Protein

➢ 200 mg Potassium

➢ 29 mg Phosphorus

What You Need:

➢ Pepper

➢ Chopped chives, 1 tsp

➢ Cauliflower, 1 head

➢ Olive oil, 1 tbsp plus more

➢ Chopped thyme, 1 tsp

What You Do:

1. Turn your oven to 400° F degrees. Use a small amount of olive oil and grease a baking sheet.
2. Place the pepper, chives, thyme, 1 tablespoon olive oil, and cauliflower. Using your hands, toss all ingredients until well coated.
3. Spread coated cauliflower onto the baking sheet.
4. Bake for 10 minutes. Take out of the oven, turn the cauliflower over, and bake for another 10 minutes for a total of 20 minutes.
5. Eat with your favorite main dish.

Chicken Meatballs

Servings: 6

Macros Per Serving:

- 85 Calories
- 67 mg Sodium
- 8 g Protein
- 200 mg Potassium
- 91 mg Phosphorus

What You Need:

- Red pepper flakes
- Pepper
- Minced garlic, 1 tsp
- Egg, 1
- Chopped scallion, 1
- Bread crumbs, .25 c
- Ground chicken, .5 lb

What You Do:

1. Turn your oven to 400° F.
2. Place red pepper flakes, pepper, garlic, egg, scallion, bread crumbs, and ground chicken into a large bowl.
3. Mix everything together using your hands
4. Form this mixture into meatballs and put them on a baking sheet.
5. Allow them to cook for 25 minutes. Flip them over several times during cooking until they are golden brown.
6. Serve and enjoy.

Chicken Salad Wraps

Servings: 4

Macros Per Serving:

- 110 Calories
- 61 mg Sodium
- 13 g Protein
- 200 mg Potassium
- 117 mg Phosphorus

What You Need:

- Large lettuce leaves, 4
- Pepper
- Mayonnaise, .25 c
- Chopped celery, 1 stalk
- Seedless red grapes, .5 c
- Chopped scallion, 1
- Cooked shredded chicken, 8 ounces

What You Do:

1. Place the mayonnaise, celery, grapes, scallion, and chicken into a bowl and mix well.
2. Sprinkle on some pepper and give another stir.
3. Take one lettuce leaf and spoon some chicken salad onto the middle.
4. Wrap the lettuce leaf around the chicken mixture.
5. Serve and enjoy.

Biscuits

Macros Per Serving:

- ➢ 190 Calories
- ➢ 45 mg Sodium
- ➢ 3 g Protein
- ➢ 126 mg Potassium
- ➢ 27 mg Phosphorus

What You Need:

- ➢ Unsweetened rice milk, .25 c
- ➢ Water, .5 c
- ➢ Lard, .5 c
- ➢ Sugar, 1 tbsp
- ➢ Phosphorus-free baking powder, 1 tbsp
- ➢ Plain flour, 2 c

What You Do:

1. Turn your oven to 350° F. Line a baking sheet with parchment.
2. Mix the flour, sugar, and baking powder into a large bowl.
3. Add in the lard and mix everything together with your fingers to incorporate the lard into the flour until coarse crumbs form. You could also use a pastry cutter if you don't like using your hands.
4. Make a well in the center of the flour. Pour in the rice milk and water. Use a fork and mix until mixture holds together into a dough. Don't over mix.

5. On a floured surface, pat the dough out until it is about a half-inch thick.

6. Cut dough into biscuits and put them onto the prepared baking sheet. You should be able to get 10 biscuits out of the dough.

7. Bake for 12 to 15 minutes. The biscuit's top should be golden.

Spritz Cookies

Servings: 12

Macros Per Serving:

- 271 Calories
- 11 mg Sodium
- 3 g Protein
- 39 mg Potassium
- 40 mg Phosphorus

What You Need:

- Plain flour, 2 c
- Vanilla, 2 tsp
- Eggs, 1
- Sugar, .5 c
- Unsalted butter, 1 c

What You Do:

1. Turn your oven to 400° F. Line a baking sheet with parchment.
2. Place sugar and room-temperature butter into a large bowl. Beat everything together with an electric mixer until fluffy and thick. This will take about 3 minutes.
3. Add in the vanilla and egg. Take a rubber spatula and scrape down the bowl. Beat just until egg is incorporated.
4. Add flour and blend on low speed until thoroughly blended.
5. Drop batter onto the prepared baking sheet using a spoon.
6. Bake 5 to 7 minutes until lightly browned and firm.
7. Remove from oven and cool completely on a wire rack.
8. Once cooled, keep it in an airtight container. This will keep about a week. Do not store in the refrigerator.

Citrusy Sesame Cookies

Servings: 18

Macros Per Serving:

➢ 150 Calories

➢ 5 mg Sodium

➢ 2 g Protein

➢ 25 mg Potassium

➢ 29 mg Phosphorus

What You Need:

➢ Orange zest, 1 tsp

➢ Baking soda, .5 tsp

➢ Lemon zest, 1 tsp

➢ Toasted sesame seeds, 2 tbsp

➢ Plain flour, 2 c

➢ Vanilla, 1 tsp

➢ Egg, 1

➢ Sugar, .5 c

➢ Unsalted butter, .75 c

What You Do:

1. Place sugar and room-temperature butter into a large bowl. Use an electric mixer and blend them together for 3 minutes.

2. Add in the vanilla and egg and blend to mix well. Scrape down the bowl with a rubber spatula.

3. Add the orange and lemon zest, baking soda, sesame seeds, and flour into a small bowl. Mix everything together.

4. Add this in the batter and mix until thoroughly blended.

5. Roll out the dough into a long cylinder that is about 2 inches in diameter. Wrap this up in Saran wrap and refrigerate for an hour.

6. While dough is firming up, turn your oven on to 350° F. Line a baking sheet with parchment.

7. Remove the chilled cookie dough and slice into half inch rounds. Place them on the baking sheet.

8. Bake them for 10 to 12 minutes. They should turn golden.

9. Place them on a wire rack to completely cool.

10. Once they are cooled, keep them in an airtight container. They will last for about a week. You could also freeze these cookies for 2 months.

Pear Chips

Servings: 4

Macros Per Serving:

- 101 Calories
- 2 mg Sodium
- 1 g Protein
- 183 mg Potassium
- 17 mg Phosphorus

What You Need:

- Sugar, 1 tbsp
- Ground cinnamon, 2 tsp
- Pears, 4
- Olive oil cooking spray

What You Do:

1. Turn your oven to 200° F. Lay parchment on a cookie sheet and coat with nonstick spray.
2. Core and cut the pears into 1/8-inch slices.
3. Place the pear slices onto the baking sheet. Make sure no pears overlap.
4. Combine the cinnamon and sugar together.
5. Sprinkle the pears with the cinnamon mixture.
6. Bake for 3 to 4 hours until chips are dry. Remove from the oven and completely cool.
7. Place into an airtight container and store in a cool dark place for about 4 days.

Guacamole with Edamame

Servings: 4

Macros Per Serving:

- 63 Calories
- 3 mg Sodium
- 3 g Protein
- 152 mg Potassium
- 48 mg Phosphorus

What You Need:

- Minced garlic, 1 tsp
- Chopped cilantro, 2 tbsp
- Zest and juice of one lemon
- Water, .25 c
- Olive oil, 1 tbsp
- Shelled, frozen edamame, 1 c

What You Do:

1. Make sure the edamame is thawed. Place it into a food processor along with garlic, olive oil, cilantro, lemon zest, lemon juice, and water.
2. Pulse until blended, but chunky.
3. Serve immediately.

Mushroom Couscous

Servings: 5

Macros Per Serving:

- 237 Calories
- 7 mg Sodium
- 8 g Protein
- 165 mg Potassium
- 115 mg Phosphorus

What You Need:

- Couscous, 10 oz
- Water, 3.5 c
- Chopped oregano, 1 tbsp
- Minced garlic, 1 tsp
- Chopped sweet onion, .25 medium
- Mixed mushrooms, 1 c
- Olive oil, 1 tbsp

What You Do:

1. Warm the oil in a large skillet.
2. Put the garlic, onion, and mushrooms into skillet and sauté for 6 minutes until tender.
3. Add in the water and oregano. Turn heat up and allow to boil.
4. Set it off the heat and add in the couscous. Stir well. Place lid on skillet and allow to stand for 5 minutes.
5. After 5 minutes, take a fork and fluff the couscous.
6. Serve and enjoy.

Collard Rolls with Peanut Sauce

Servings: 8

Macros Per Serving:

- 174 Calories
- 42 mg Sodium
- 8 g Protein
- 284 mg Potassium
- 56 mg Phosphorus

What You Need:

- For the Dipping Sauce:
- Red chili flakes, .25 tsp
- Juice of a lime
- Honey, 2 tbsp
- Peanut butter, .25 c
- For the Salad Rolls:
- Bean sprouts, 1 c
- Thinly sliced purple cabbage, 1 c
- Bunch collard greens
- Extra-firm tofu, 4 oz
- Cilantro leaves and stems, .5 c
- Carrots sliced into matchsticks, 2

What You Do:

1. To make the dipping sauce, add the chili flakes, lime juice, honey, and peanut butter to a food processor. Combine the mixture until

it becomes smooth. Mix in 2 tablespoons of water to reach your desired consistency.

2. For the salad rolls: press all of the excess moisture out of the tofu. Slice them into ½-inch thick matchsticks.

3. Get rid of the tough stems from the collards and place to the side.

4. Cup a collard green leaf in one hand and add a couple of strips of tofu and a small bit of cabbage, carrots, and bean sprouts. Top with a sprig of cilantro and roll up. Place the roll, seam-side down, on a platter. Continue with the rest of the rolls.

5. Serve the rolls along with the dipping sauce.

Roasted Mint Carrots

Servings: 6

Macros Per Serving:

- 51 Calories
- 52 mg Sodium
- 1 g Protein
- 242 mg Potassium
- 26 mg Phosphorus

What You Need:

- Thinly sliced mint, .25 c
- Pepper
- EVOO, 1 tbsp
- Trimmed carrots, 1 lb

What You Do:

1. Set your oven to 350° F.
2. Lay the carrots out on a baking sheet and coat them with the olive oil. Shake the carrots around so that they are coated with oil. Season with some pepper.
3. Let them bake for 20 minutes, or until they are browned and tender. Stir twice while they are cooking.
4. Sprinkle the top with mint.

Spanish Potatoes

Servings: 3

Macros Per Serving:

- ➢ 92 Calories
- ➢ 21 mg Sodium
- ➢ 1 g Protein
- ➢ 271 mg Potassium
- ➢ 34 mg Phosphorus

What You Need:

- ➢ Low-fat sour cream, 1 tbsp
- ➢ Smoked paprika, 1 tbsp
- ➢ Lemon, .5
- ➢ Chopped parsley, 1 tbsp
- ➢ Sweet potatoes, 2
- ➢ EVOO, 1 tbsp

What You Do:

1. Peel and dice the sweet potatoes.
2. Boil the potatoes for 10 minutes. Drain the water off. Add the potatoes to a fresh pot of boil water and boil for 10 more minutes.
3. Meanwhile, heat the oil to high.
4. Add in the potatoes and sprinkle with paprika. Sauté for 15 minutes.
5. Serve, tossed in the lemon juice, fresh herbs, and topped with sour cream.

Coleslaw

Servings: 2

Macros Per Serving:

- 89 Calories
- 30 mg Sodium
- 1 g Protein
- 208 mg Potassium
- 25 mg Phosphorus

What You Need:

- EVOO, 1 tbsp
- Chopped parsley, 1 tbsp
- Sliced cabbage, 1 c
- Zest and juice of a lemon
- Sliced carrot

What You Do:

1. Mix all of the ingredients together.
2. Chill before serving.

Mashed Rutabaga and Turnip

Servings: 2

Macros Per Serving:

➢ 103 Calories

➢ 23 mg Sodium

➢ 2 g Protein

➢ 364 mg Potassium

➢ 56 mg Phosphorus

What You Need:

➢ Pepper

➢ Chopped turnips, 2

➢ EVOO, 1 tbsp

➢ Chopped tarragon, 2 tbsp

➢ Chopped rutabaga, .75 c

What You Do:

1. Boil the turnip and rutabaga in a pot of water for 15 to 20 minutes. They should be very soft.
2. Drain and mix in the olive oil and tarragon, and some pepper.
3. Mashup to your desired consistency and serve.

Conclusion

Thank you for making it through to the end of Renal Diet Cookbook. I hope that it has been informative and will help you to reach your goals, no matter what they may be.

Just because you have been diagnosed with CKD doesn't mean you are doomed for dialysis. With a few changes to your diet, you can prevent dialysis and slow or stop the progress of your kidney disease. As you have learned, your diet can be delicious and healthy. The important thing to remember is to watch your proteins, phosphorus, potassium, and sodium.

Don't wait any longer! Change your diet and help your kidneys.

CPSIA information can be obtained
at www.ICGtesting.com
Printed in the USA
BVHW022118050223
657818BV00007B/598

9 781774 340431